Mushrooms
for
Health

{ *Medicinal
Secrets of
Northeastern
Fungi*

GREG A. MARLY

Down East Books

ANY SERIOUS WRITING PROJECT requires a concentrated focus of time, energy, and resources by the author. This is doubly true for *Mushrooms for Health*, my first book-length project. I am deeply grateful and indebted to my family for supporting me through the process and helping create the incubator for this book. *Mushrooms for Health* is dedicated to Valli and Dash in grateful reminder of their patience, humor, and exasperated goodwill as I filled their lives with medicinal mushroom lore, stacks of papers, bushels of drying mushrooms, and gallons of unexpected decoctions. They remain my fiercest defenders and most realistic critics.

This book has also benefited from the mushrooming insight and keen eye of my friend and fellow mushroomer, Michaeline Mulvey.

Disclaimer

The practice of mushroom identification requires study and good resources. Although this book gives information needed to identify the medicinal mushroom species described here, it is not intended as a general guide for mushroom identification, and it may not specifically include all relevant and established safe practices. Please consult an expert or obtain the necessary education before collecting and eating any wild mushrooms. Down East Books and Down East Enterprise, Inc., its agents, officers and employees, and the author, accept no responsibility for injuries or damages that may result from information, or the interpretation of such, herein.

This book is intended as an information and resource guide for practitioners and end users of medicinal mushrooms. It is based upon a compilation of the worldwide available research on medicinal mushrooms. The statements made in this book have not been evaluated by the Food and Drug Administration. Medicinal mushroom supplements are not intended to diagnose, treat, cure, or prevent any disease. If you are concerned about your health, please consult a trusted health professional before beginning any new plan of care.

Down East Books

An imprint of The Globe Pequot Publishing Group, Inc.
64 South Main Street
Essex, CT 06426
www.globepequot.com

Library of Congress Cataloging-in-Publication Data

Marley, Greg A., 1955-
Mushrooms for health: medicinal secrets of Northeastern fungi/ Greg A. Marley.
    p. cm.
Includes bibliographical references and index.
ISBN 978-0-89272-808-4
1. F ungi – Therapeutic use. 2. Mushrooms – Therapeutic use. 3. Mushrooms – Northeastern States – Identification. I. Title.

RS165.F72M37 2009
615.9'5296 – dc22

2009031306

Contents

Introduction

Ith regard to the use of medicinal mushrooms and the overall appreciation
of wild mushrooms, America finds itself in a timely convergence of curiosity,
interest, and need.

We live in a mycophobic, or mushroom-fearing, culture, assuming that any
wild mushroom is deadly until proven otherwise, in spite of the reality that far
less than 1 percent of wild mushrooms hold the potential to kill. For the past ten
years, I have served as a volunteer consultant with the Northern New England Poi-
son Control Center, assisting with mushroom identification in suspected poison-
mushroom ingestion cases. Fully 80 percent of the mushroom-related calls in New
England and nationally involve a young, "grazer-age" preschool child without any
symptom of distress. In most cases, a parent or other family member found the
child with a mushroom in hand or mouth and feared the worst. Very few of these
cases result in any significant illness. The common emergency room response has
been, at the least, to administer charcoal or induce vomiting. One can be sure that
any child who did not fear mushrooms before the event certainly did afterward.

In recent years, Americans began to embrace the opportunities presented
by the wild mushrooms growing in our midst. Many people attending a talk on
wild mushrooms relate fond tales from their childhood of collecting mushrooms
with a parent, grandparent, or aunt from the "old country." They mourn the loss
of the knowledge of things wild and the connection to the traditions of their
heritage. Some people focus on the rich array of edible mushrooms whose flavors
so outshine the pale mushrooms easily available in the produce section of our
supermarkets. These edible-only enthusiasts will, at times, wish to know only if
the specimen being examined is good to eat or not. Others seek to increase their
understanding of the natural world around them and the role fungi play in this
world. Often they are building on a base of knowledge they already use in their
lives. And now more people are turning to the rich and diverse world of fungi to
assist with maintaining, or returning to, optimal health.

In many of the traditionally mycophillic (mushroom-loving) cultures of the
world, mushrooms have long been a valued source of both food and medicine.
In China and Japan, Ling Chi, or Reishi (*Ganoderma lucidum*) has been viewed as
a panacea worthy of royalty. There is an often-told story of Japanese mushroom

collectors who so valued Maitake *(Grifola frondosa)*, as both a food source and a health tonic that they might go to the grave before divulging the locations of their Maitake trees. As the story is told, even as death neared, only the eldest or favored son would learn the secret.

The integration of mushrooms in the cultures of China, Japan, Korea, and many of the countries of eastern and northern Europe has led scientists in those countries to take the lead in researching the medicinal uses of the mushrooms long used in traditional folk medicine. The addition of mushrooms into the diet in Traditional Chinese Medicine (TCM) is in recognition of the added benefits and immune-protective effects they have in balancing the life force, or qi, of the body. As modern research has sought to understand the protective effects of medicinal mushrooms, we recognized the immune-boosting potential of the polysaccharide component in some species. As we have sought to understand the traditional use of mushrooms such as Reishi and Chaga in managing inflammatory response in the body, we have begun to learn that many of the terpene sterols in these mushrooms reduce inflammation.

The same has held true in the antimicrobial actions of some mushrooms and fungal components. The exploration of the penicillin mold as a possible source of antibiotics followed a series of initial observations that mold inhibited the growth of bacteria. Observations that perennial and other long-lived mushroom fruiting bodies seem resistant to bacterial attack led to the exploration of antimicrobial compounds in these species.

In many other parts of the world, medicinal mushrooms, mushroom extracts, or partially purified fractions extracted from mushrooms or mycelia are considered front-line medications and used in the treatment of various forms of cancers and other disorders. But the United States has a much longer and more intense vetting process for approval of a new drug, a process that takes, on average, more than seven years and costs in excess of $800 million for the clinical trials and other testing. As a result, only those products seen as clinically effective *and* likely to repay the associated research and development costs enter the clinical testing stream. Meanwhile, many of these same mushrooms and mushroom extracts can be used as dietary supplements by informed consumers interested in accessing their health-promoting benefits.

In spite of the fact that the United States spends more on health care and medical research than any other country in the world, we have been very slow to embrace the potential of mushrooms as aids to healthy living. A culture that does not embrace the use of wild mushrooms as food will certainly be slow to embrace them as medicine. Yet the change is happening. The public is hungry to take steps to enable them to feel more in control of health care and the use of health-care dollars. After a generation of "food as indulgence," we are increasingly aware of the connection between diet and health. The epidemic in obesity, and the associated surge in the rates of childhood-onset diabetes and other weight-related illnesses, has fueled a growing need to eat more fresh, less-processed food. The concept of functional foods is filtering into our consciousness as we improve our awareness of the importance of diet. If we know that a good-tasting fresh food packs an added punch as a health-promoting dietary aid, then all the more reason to find room for such foods in our weekly meal menus.

One physician I know urges his patients, overweight or not, to concentrate their food shopping on the perimeter aisles of the store where the fresh food is displayed, and to venture into the center aisles of snack food, junk food, and carbohydrate-heavy processed foods only as absolutely needed. Unfortunately for those on a limited budget, eating fresh is more costly; for those with busy lives and crowded schedules, cooking fresh food takes more time. Yet the payout is great as we take more responsibility for good health.

The promise of medicinal mushrooms lies in their role as one step in a healthy diet and as a component of a healthy lifestyle. The health-promoting compounds in mushrooms—be they beta glucans, triterpenes, or other components—offer the possibility of improved bodily functioning. They are not a panacea. A diet of medicinal mushrooms and Twinkies is not a healthy diet. But integrating medicinal mushrooms as a supplement into an otherwise healthy diet can add additional support to your health and maybe balance out the occasional indulgence in less healthy, but tasty, food.

The northeastern states are home to many of the world's most researched and clinically supported medicinal mushrooms. With a little effort to learn about mushrooms, and at the cost of a healthy hike in the woods, you can start to collect your own mushrooms. Adding them to your diet requires little in the way of training. Alternatively, after reading this book, you can choose to seek out medicinal mushroom products from a reliable source and reap their benefits without needing to collect your own. My hope is that in the following pages you will find a reason to take another step along the road to mycophillia.

Chapter 1

How to Use This Book

Mushrooms for Heath is an invitation—an invitation to bring mushrooms into your life as functional, health-promoting food. As you read this material and consider the possible benefits of adding mushrooms to your diet, I invite you to allow yourself to blur the distinction between food and medicine.

Most Americans grow up learning to distrust and fear mushrooms. We are raised believing that wild mushrooms are probably deadly, and that even handling one places us at risk of being poisoned. I hear the reflection of these beliefs each time I speak to people about mushrooms: "Are they poisonous to touch?" "How can I get rid of the mushrooms that grow on my lawn?" We see the annual crop of wild mushrooms growing in our yards not as potential meals or even as representations of the creative beauty of nature but rather as invasive organisms with suspect intentions. From that place of fear we plot how to rid our kingdom of the invaders.

Many Americans trace their ancestry back to cultures and lands where mushrooms are passionately embraced and regarded as a much-loved and valued source of food, a resource for tonics to aid in health maintenance, and a source of medicine in times of need. In these mycophillic lands, mushrooms are learned from the cradle, and a child reaches school age knowing many species and having taken an active role in collecting with the family. In Russia, for instance, nursery rhymes teach the names and descriptions of some of the common species. Fairy and folk tales incorporate mushrooms into myth and legend and become beloved children's stories. Yet, in the assimilation of immigrants into the melting pot that is America, many have lost touch with this vibrant part of their cultures. My mother is of French and German stock, and it is only in the last ten years that I learned that she, as a child, collected mushrooms with her mother on their sheep ranch in Montana. By the time she was a parent raising her own children in New Mexico, mushrooms rarely appeared on our dinner table and only did so in the guise of Campbell's Cream of Mushroom Soup or some similarly domesticated and disguised form. My father, of firmly mycophobic Irish heritage, saw to it that mushrooms never graced the Marley table in any recognizable form. The stories of my mother's family collecting Pink Bottoms in the summer, or Morels in the spring, was never a part of the family lore I learned as I grew up. Yet somehow I made a leap into the world of mushrooming. As an avid amateur mycologist and mushroom educator bringing the world of mushrooms to hundreds of people each year, I see the interest rising in people seeking to reintegrate mushrooms into their lives.

Mushrooms for Health contains species-specific and general information about the collection, preservation, preparation, and use of medicinal mushrooms. It is designed to help you locate, identify, and use the more common and well-researched medicinal mushrooms found in the northeastern United States. In order to better understand the beneficial effect of medicinal mushrooms on our bodies, I have included a chapter devoted to a basic understanding of the human immune system and a chapter on how mushrooms interact with the body. I urge you to read these chapters carefully and then to refer to them for a better understanding of how different mushroom constituents are helpful when used as dietary supplements.

The second section of the book is devoted to a review of the common and accepted medicinal species found growing in the Northeast. In each chapter I will present information including:

- Description of the mushroom as an aid in identification
- Time of occurrence, fruiting habits, and frequency
- The mushroom's ecological role and place in the environment
- History and tradition of their medicinal and culinary use
- Commercial medicinal applications and products, where available
- Recommendations for collection, preparation, preservation, and use
- Recent and current research and clinical results supporting their medicinal use

This book presents a condensed synopsis of the strongest evidence supporting the use of medicinal mushrooms for health promotion. As more countries discover the potential of medicinal mushrooms, scientists have increasingly carried out research on their utilization. Much of the initial research has been carried out using animal and human cell lines in vitro or on laboratory animals. Only later have mushroom products been tested using human subjects, and this clinical research remains lacking for many species. The knowledge gained through years of experimentation will be reviewed for each species, and information on their traditional and current use as medicinal aids will be presented as simply and cleanly as possible. A brief glossary of mycological and medicinal terminology is included to help the reader understand any scientific and medical language. The medical

Timing Is Everything

Whether you are seeking medicinal mushrooms to address a health concern or to use as a general tonic and preventive strategy, having an adequate supply will, sooner or later, become a concern. Most species fruit in a relatively narrow window of time, so it is important to harvest and preserve a quantity of mushrooms when they are at hand.

Only after they have built up sufficient food and energy reserves will adequate rainfall and the proper temperature induce these fungi to fruit. In New England, that means most species fruit in the late summer or autumn. This is especially true for fleshy species such as Oyster Mushrooms and Maitake, which must be collected when they are available, usually a week or so after a significant rain. (Woody polypores like the Artist's Conk have a more extended period of activity and, because of the stability of their host, are less dependent on rain.)

As I write these words, it is October 27, and the fall Oyster Mushroom *(Pleurotus ostreatus)* is fruiting in all its glory. I have no doubt that I can collect twenty pounds of prime Oyster Mushrooms and will be faced with the happy dilemma of how to preserve their goodness, using a combination of drying or cooking and freezing. I know the benefits certainly will be worth the time spent.

portion is heavily weighted toward an understanding of immune system terminology. For those who would like information about the research supporting the use of medicinal mushrooms, I have included an extensive bibliography of references, including some excellent review articles.

Mushrooms for Health is not a comprehensive guide for mushroom identification. Though it will address common look-alike species, it is not meant to take the place of a more complete field guide to area mushrooms and should not be used as a basis for learning mushroom identification skills. Please refer to "References" (page 132) for a list of recommended field guides and Internet resources for mushroom identification. I strongly recommend that a novice mushroomer take a class on mushroom identification or go out with someone who knows the major species and can act as a guide. There are a number of mushroom clubs and mycological associations scattered around the Northeast. Consider joining one to gain access to other mushroom enthusiasts. Mycology is one area of learning where a mentor can be invaluable as an aid for reality-testing and the building of familiarity and confidence. Though a picture can indeed be worth a thousand words, a living example seen in the natural environment or the hands of a knowledgeable local guide is irreplaceable. In the United States, one of the largest impediments

My Evolution as a Mushroomer

When I was fifteen, I traveled for the first time from New Mexico to the eastern United States. I left behind a climate of high desert with an average annual rainfall of less than nine inches and spent the summer in Rhinebeck, New York, amidst the rolling hills and lush woods of the mid–Hudson River Valley. New York state averages almost five times the annual precipitation of New Mexico, and I knew I was in a different world when, early on the third morning of the trip, I awoke to a world of dense, verdant hillsides in western Pennsylvania. I spent four summers in New York state between 1971 and 1980, much of that time in the eastern deciduous forest.

As a teenager, I had been struck by the beauty and uniqueness of wild mushrooms. In 1973, I picked up my first mushroom field guide, a Dover reprint of Louis Krieger's 1936 *Mushroom Handbook*, and began to explore the fascinating group of colorful moss-dwellers called fungi.

I was also interested in foraging for wild foods, and I spent hours in the woods with my Euell Gibbons guides, stalking the wild asparagus and other uncultivated foods. It was, therefore, no surprise that my interest in wild mushrooms broadened into the possibilities of mushrooms as food. My progress was slow because I had no mentor who knew the mushrooms and could guide me. Being a cautious adventurer, and using field guides and curiosity, I slowly began to learn the more common groups of mushrooms, both the edibles and the poisonous, and to collect the most common edibles.

The first mushroom I ate was a Puffball growing under the apple trees in my parents' yard in Albuquerque. It was in the fall of 1973, and the rains had brought out a flush of these small, whitish, baseball-sized fungi. I followed Krieger's wisdom about the genus Calvatia: "The beginner is advised to start with these Puffballs in risking his life in the cause of mycophagy. But there is no risk, for they are all both safe and good to eat so long as the flesh is white, dry and compact."

The following year I added *Agaricus campestris*, Meadow Mushroom, to my list of edibles, collecting these from the sprinkler-watered and manure-enriched ball fields at the University of New Mexico campus where I attended undergraduate classes. In 1977 I took my first class in mycology at UNM. That autumn I found a massive flush of *Coprinus comatus*, Shaggy Manes, fruiting on campus. For three years, each late fall I collected large quantities of the young, firm Shaggy Manes as they emerged from the soil and learned just how delicate and tasty they are sautéed in butter or as the main character in a simple cream soup.

It's easy in hindsight to appreciate the slow process of adding new mushrooms to my list of edible species. Seven years after I first bought a mushroom guide, I had eaten three species. In the late 1970s, New Mexico did not have a mycological society or any other mushrooming club, and I was not aware of anyone other than me out collecting mushrooms. Only after moving to Maine in 1980 did I begin to connect with other mushroom hunters and to develop a small community of mushrooming enthusiasts with whom to share information and excitement.

to starting to collect and use wild mushrooms is developing a healthy mix of competence and confidence. A good field guide can build intellectual competence, a knowledgeable guide, confidence.

The good news is that most of the species of medicinal mushrooms addressed in this book are easy to distinguish and do not resemble any dangerously toxic species. In general, no poisonous polypore fungi are found growing on wood, and many of our better-known medicinal species are wood-degrading polypores. A word of caution: I have heard people attempt to make this statement apply to all mushrooms growing on wood, not just polypores. Some gilled mushrooms that grow on wood are quite toxic, including one known as the Deadly Galerina. That said, you must always be 100 percent confident in your identification of the mushroom before using it for food or as a dietary supplement.

Another piece of good news comes in the guise of advice. I did not learn all the edible and toxic mushrooms in the woods before I started eating wild mushrooms. Over time, I learned a few edible and easily identified species, and I began to integrate them into my diet as I became confident in my ability to identify them. I suggest the same path for bringing medicinal and/or edible mushrooms into your life. Mycophagy, the use of mushrooms as food, should not be viewed as an extreme sport where the goal is to compete for the greatest number of species consumed. The pursuit of the longest "life list" (as birders refer to this notion) when collecting edible mushrooms is fraught with risk. It becomes a slippery slope that leads to eating ever more questionable or little-known species and increases the likelihood of mushroom sickening or poisoning. I know many satisfied mushroomers and mushroom eaters with decades of experience who happily collect and consume only two or three types that they feel comfortable knowing.

If you follow a similar path with medicinal mushrooms, you will be certain to have a positive experience. Learn the common medicinal mushrooms growing in your area and, as you do so, begin to integrate them into your life. Eat Oyster Mushrooms in the spring and fall, make Chaga tea in the cold evenings of winter—but only when you feel confident in your identification of the species. I recently received an e-mail response to a survey I conducted about the species of wild mushrooms consumed by people in New England. This respondent reported that she has eaten the same two kinds of mushrooms for fifty years. She learned them as a child, from a relative, and does not know their Latin or common name, only their Italian name. She did write that she would be interested in learning about a few more species she can eat.

Anyone writing about a topic as extensive as "mushrooms for health" has to make decisions about the number of species to include. My aim is to cover the mushrooms likely to be found growing naturally in the northeastern United States and Eastern Canada that have some history of medicinal use or a notable level of research supporting their use as medicinals. In addition, these are mushrooms that are relatively easy to collect and prepare for use.

There are other mushrooms in use medicinally worldwide and supported by good research that I do not include for the simple reason that they are not found in the Northeast. These include Shiitake (*Lentinula edodes*), Royal Sun Agaricus *(Agaricus blazei)*, Cordyceps (*Cordyceps sinensis*), and Mesima (*Phellinus linteus*). I also left out Split Gill (*Schizophyllum commune*), as the medicinal use of this species is based upon use of cultivated mycelium only, not the fruiting body. I have little doubt that additional species of common forest mushrooms will be added to the ranks of medicinals in coming years. Testing on a wide number of species continues around the world, and each month brings additional information to whet the appetite.

I am regularly asked about the medicinal benefits of the hallucinogenic mushrooms in the psilocybin group and the Fly Agaric (*Amanita muscaria*). Although psilocybin has shown some benefit in addressing symptoms of anxiety and depression in carefully designed settings, I chose to not pursue that particular application of medicinal mushrooms in these pages. A treatment of this fascinating topic will be included in a future book project.

Chapter 2

What Is a Mushroom?

A mushroom is the fruiting body of a fungus, one large enough to be easily seen with the naked eye. Mushrooms take on many forms: The classic round-domed cap with an intricate set of radiating gills on a central stalk growing on the ground (or aseptically wrapped in plastic in the produce section of your nearby supermarket), is what most people hold in their minds. Other growth forms include the round spheres of Puffballs; the shallow, dish-like cup fungi; coral-like aggregations; pitted Morels; the fleshy polypore Boletes; woody shelves; brackets; and conks such as Reishi. The mushroom is analogous to an apple or any other fruit from a plant. Its reason for existence is to produce, display, and distribute the seeds of the next generation. And, just like the apple hanging from the tree, the mushroom is a very small portion of the whole fungal body. Where the entire apple vegetative body is composed of the roots, branches, twigs, and leaves, as well as the fruit, the fungus too has a vegetative body. In the case of the mushroom, the vegetative body is generally not visible, so it would be easy to believe that the visible part is the entire organism. This is not the case. Let's look at the Oyster Mushroom as an example.

When we find the eruption of multiple fleshy caps fruiting in a cluster on an old sugar maple in late October, we are seeing the end result of a great deal of life work by *Pleurotus ostreatus,* the species name for what we call the Oyster Mushroom. Life for our cluster of Oyster Mushrooms began when a spore, the microscopic "seed" of *P. ostreatus,* landed in a wound on the maple tree trunk, found the proper amount of moisture and warmth, and germinated. The germinating spore developed into a microscopic thread of **hyphae,*** which form the basis of the vegetative growth of the fungus. (Most people know hyphae as the cotton-like fuzz they find on bread left too long wrapped in plastic in their breadbox.) These hyphal threads grow through the substrate, colonizing the heartwood of the sugar maple, and as they elongate, they produce enzymes that break down the lignins and cellulose in the wood of the tree. These very powerful enzymes flow out of the cell and into the surrounding environment, where they break down the complex carbohydrate cellulose and lignin into simple sugars that are brought back into the cell as food. In this way, the fungus can be said to literally eat its way through its host, with the heartwood the main course.

*This and other words in boldface throughout the book are further defined in the Glossary (page 130).

Mushroom Names, Common and Formal

Every known living thing has a name, and most have several. The scientific name is made up of two words, the first referring to the genus and the second to the species. A genus is a group of related organisms sharing a number of common features. Organisms within a species are able to produce viable offspring that breed true to the qualities defining the species. As an example, the mushroom *Cantharellus cibarius*, known commonly as the Chanterelle, is a member of the genus *Cantharellus*, and is the species *cibarius*. Using the genus and species name, I can talk about the Chanterelle with any mushroomer the world over or look it up on a Web site, in a scientific journal article, or in a field guide written in any language.

The common name for *C. cibarius* (in repeated references to a mushroom, the genus is abbreviated to the first letter) changes frequently, depending upon where you are and what language you are speaking. Even within one country, a well-known and useful mushroom may have a number of common names. In a recent monograph, Pilz et al. (2003) compiled a list of more than ninety common names in twenty-five languages for *C. cibarius* and felt certain that the list was not comprehensive. One difficulty with Chanterelle as a common name is that it is also used informally to refer to any species of mushroom belonging to the genus *Cantharellus*.

In the context of this book, mushrooms will be referred to in a mixture of their scientific names and their most widely accepted or known common name. In the case of Chaga *(Inonotus obliquus)* and Reishi *(Ganoderma lucidum)*, the best-known of their common medicinal names come from other countries and languages. In all cases, the goal is to be clear about names without being needlessly complex.

Cellulose, along with lignins and other compounds, makes up the cell walls of plants and are the basic foodstuff for a host of **saprobic** fungi. The fungal enzymes, excreted into the environment surrounding the hyphal cells, begin the process of breaking down the complex building blocks of the wood into smaller sugars that can enter the fungal cells and be further broken down to release their energy and basic nutrients. Through this process, carbon dioxide is released into the atmosphere and nutrients are utilized by the fungus or made available to other plants and organisms in the area. Thus is nutrient recycling facilitated between the dead tree and the next generations of living organisms.

Without fungi, bacteria, and protozoa fulfilling the role of decomposers for the world, dead plant and animal matter would build up on the forest floor, the available nutrients in the soil would be tied up in dead tissue, and the photosynthetic machine would quickly grind to a halt as plants became starved for the essential minerals nitrogen, potassium, phosphorus, and other elements. No other class of organisms can decompose dead plant tissue as efficiently as the fungi. They have evolved in lockstep with the plants to be the expert undertakers. For the Oyster Mushroom and other primary saprobic fungi, cellulose and/or lignins are food. Unlike green plants, which, as autotrophs, use their chlorophyll to manufacture food from nutrients, carbon dioxide, and the sun, mushrooms are known as heterotrophs, organisms unable to make their own food but feeding on other plants or animals. We humans too are heterotrophs.

In the case of the Oyster Mushroom, as the hyphae grow through the maple heartwood, they are colonizing it. The colony of hyphae formed in this process is known as mycelium. The mycelial mat supports the growing fungus through storage of nutrients and water, transport of nutrients within the organism, and, as the conditions are right, formation of the mushroom fruiting body. In most mushrooms, fungal sex must occur before this can happen. This fleeting moment happens when the haploid hyphae originating from one spore meet and combine with the hyphae of another compatible strain of the same species. This doubles the genetic material in the cell, and after this blissful moment, the fungus is capable of forming a sexual fruiting body, the mushroom. The combined (diploid) mycelium continues to grow as it colonizes its food source, whether that is organic matter in the soil, heartwood, or pine cone, and expands the mycelial network. When the fungus has gained enough food energy, and when the conditions of temperature, moisture, and light (some fungi require specific levels of light to fruit) are conducive, the mycelia will begin to form thick **hyphal knots,** the precursors to the actual mushroom.

Our Oyster Mushroom requires low levels of light to set fruit. Consider the adaptive reason for this. If the mycelium that colonized the maple heartwood produced a mushroom deep in an enclosed cavity in the log, one that had no access to the outside air, the resulting spores would never be launched into the wind for dispersal to another site. Therefore, low levels of light would signal the mycelium that it is near the open air, but not in direct sunlight. The expanding mushroom would be out in the open, but not in the drying sun.

We live with the mystery of mushrooms appearing fully developed in our lawns and gardens seemingly overnight. Indeed, there are a number of smaller fragile mushrooms, such as the strikingly beautiful *Coprinus pliacatus,* the Parasol Inky Caps, that appear fully formed on our lawns and paths early in the morning, only to dry out and wither in the afternoon sun. They are able to grow so rapidly because, in the compact button stage, all the cells of the mature mushroom are already present. Water uptake from the mycelium rapidly fills out these compacted cells. As the mushroom expands, any object in the path of expansion will either be pushed aside or, if firm enough, deform the growing mushroom. This "pushing aside" can exert great power, as evidenced by cases of asphalt paving being broken open by expanding mushrooms.

Within a very few hours, in some species, the button, which has been forming quietly out of sight for several days, expands into maturity and begins to release its crop of spores into the air. In reality, most mushrooms require several days to reach maturity and will continue to mature and release spores for a number of days if the weather conditions remain moist.

The fruiting bodies of some species mature more slowly. The emerging buttons of Chanterelles take many days to mature in their moist, protected forest habitats—a reality I have noted often as I wait impatiently for a favorite patch to reach a size and stage where I don't feel like a cradle-robber when I pick them. Pilz's monograph on Chanterelles (Pilz, et al, 2003) notes that a Chanterelle fruiting body lives, on average, forty-five days, and some in excess of ninety days, before succumbing to decay. Some of the leathery and woody polypore bracket fungi, such as Reishi, grow slowly throughout much of the summer, releasing billions of spores in late summer or early fall. Others in this group of polypores are true perennials, adding a new layer of pores during each favorable growing period in a lifespan that can extend over decades. The Artist's Conk, fruiting on large maples, can sometimes attain a diameter exceeding two feet.

Though mushrooms are often ephemeral, the mycelial network of the fungus continues to live on, busily rotting its host substrate for as long as the food source is available. For the Maitake, a saprobe and parasite living on the heartwood of a large oak tree, the mycelium can survive for decades. I know of one tree that has regularly produced Maitake clusters since 1983 and may have been doing so for years before I found it.

Other mushrooms live out their life in a universe as small as a pine cone or the cup of an acorn and will complete their lifecycle in a matter of days or weeks as they rot their host and produce the few tiny fruiting bodies they have the life energy, or biomass, to support. These are examples of saprobes, those species of fungi with a life strategy of rotting plant matter.

A host of other fungi have enormous value as much-desired edible mushrooms, and even more value as contributors to the health of our forests. These species are known as **mycorrhizal** mushrooms, and they form symbiotic partnerships with trees, shrubs, and other plants through long-term associations with their roots. Both parties benefit from the partnership: The tree utilizes the mycelial network of the fungus as an extended root zone, able to locate and transport nutrients to the tree from a far greater distance than the traditional plant root zone; and the mushroom benefits from the donation of sugars from the tree. In a healthy forest, an individual tree might form these fungal root associations with several different mushroom species, and an individual fungus might have associations with several to many trees simultaneously. In this fashion, mature trees are even able to provide nutrition to small tree seedlings through the communication network of the fungal intermediary. Paul Stamets has written extensively about these mycelial "Internets," and I recommend his groundbreaking book *Mycelium Running* as a source of more information.

In much the same way that the saprobic Maitake growing on oak heartwood can live and produce massive quantities of fruit for many years, so the mycorrhizal species benefit from a stable food source. You don't normally see massive fruiting flushes from mycorrhizal species most years, but you can generally count on some fruiting in the same location whenever the environmental conditions are optimal. For me, it means that I always know where to find the summer's first crop of Chanterelles after the first good rains of July. As a mycorrhizal species, the Chanterelle mycelium lives perennially with the host trees.

Most mushrooms are quite delicate, somewhat in the same way that human beings are delicate, being made of up to 90 percent water and quite fleshy. In addition, they are filled with nutrients, containing up to 40 percent protein by dry weight, a small percent of lipids and fats, and many essential vitamins and minerals. This makes them a healthy food source for a host of mammals, insects, bacteria, and other fungi, so it is no surprise that mushrooms have evolved a host of chemical and structural defenses, including antibacterial agents, toxins, and tough exteriors, to protect themselves. It also makes sense that the woody "perennial" fruiting bodies, being more stable in time and place, might have several levels of protective chemicals to offer defense against predation over the years of their life. Some of these protective chemicals have medicinal value for human predators of mushrooms. Others are responsible for the occasional mushroom poisoning that can happen when people eat a mushroom species they shouldn't. Mushroom poisonings can range from a mild stomachache or gastrointestinal distress to liver failure and death. Fortunately, severe poisonings are rare in the United States. On average, one or two people a year die from mushroom poisoning in this country, as compared to an average of ninety a year who die from lightning strikes.

Mushrooms drop or forcibly eject their spores into the air, and the spores are then carried away by the slightest of breezes to land wherever they fall. The remote possibility of being deposited in a suitable environment for growth is why mushrooms, like many stationary marine organisms (think mussels or corals), make so many potential offspring and literally cast them into the wind. An individual mushroom spore is microscopically small, generally less than 20 micrometers. To put this into perspective, 100 micrometers is approximately one-tenth the thickness of a dime. In general, it requires more than 2,000 spores, lined up, to span an inch. A large mushroom can produce millions of spores every hour in its maturity. One estimate regarding *Ganoderma applanatum,* the Artist's Conk, is that a large fruiting body may produce up to 350,000 spores per second and can produce spores over a period of several months during a growing season and live for ten or more years (Hudler, 1998). Some fungi can produce spores asexually, but sexual reproduction increases genetic diversity and an organism's ability to adapt to a changing universe. Some of the macro-fungi addressed in this book may reproduce through both asexual and sexual means, but when a mushroom is produced, it is the result of sexual reproduction.

Most mycologists agree that there are approximately fourteen thousand named species of mushrooms in the world, and all will agree that there are many more to be discovered and named. This wave of discovery is very active in tropical environments but is also ongoing in temperate regions, including New England, as we expand our awareness of the diversity of fungi. It is widely reported that 5 to 10 percent of mushroom species are toxic, and 10 to 20 percent are edible. Estimates vary, in part, because of the way we define poisonous and the limits of our knowledge. *The Dictionary of Edible Mushrooms* (Chandra, 1989) reports that there are almost seven hundred known and named edible mushrooms in use in various countries of the world. Eric Boa, in his 2004 FAO report, "Wild Edible Fungi: A Global Overview of Their Use and Importance to People," collected reports on the edibility of 1,154 species from 85 countries through the use of regional sources and guides. Though testing and exploration continue, there are at least 650 species of higher fungi that have been shown to have immune-stimulating polysaccharides in their tissues. But the vast majority of these have not been well studied. We have barely begun to explore the possibilities offered by the world of mushrooms.

Chapter 3

Mushrooms and Our Health

In 1991, hikers along the Austrian and Italian borders of the Alps came upon the pre-served body of a Neolithic man freshly melted out of glacier ice. We now know from radioisotope tests done on the body and artifacts found with it that Ötzi, the Iceman, as he came to be called, walked this earth about 5,300 years ago. Among the artifacts found with the body were two fungi, a find rarely, if ever, associated with preserved bodies and therefore significant. *Fomes fomentarius*, the Tinder Conk or Amadou, was found in the form of pounded or shredded fruiting bodies almost filling a leather satchel. Two examples of *Piptoporus betulinus*, the Birch Polypore, were found dried, shaped, and threaded through leather straps and worn around his neck. Though we may never know the reason these two fungi were carried by the Iceman, and scientists continue to debate their significance (Poder, 2005), several attributes of these two spe-cies may relate to this question and help provide answers.

The Tinder Conk has long been valued as an effective means to catch a spark from flint or the friction-produced heat of a bow drill and ignite a fire. It has also been utilized to transport the glowing embers of the fire to the next campsite. Many examples of these arts are continued today by practitioners of the primitive arts of survival (Storm, 2004). Clearly these skills were of life-preserving significance to a man traveling in the high mountains at the end of the last Ice Age. The dry, shred-ded fruiting body of the Tinder Conk has also been used on wounds to stanch bleed-ing by many native peoples around the world (Gyozo, 2005, and Hobbs, 1995), and recent studies of the mushroom show broad antimicrobial properties that would support the use for healing wounds beyond the mechanical use as a wound dress-ing. Could the Iceman have had knowledge of this?

Birch Polypore has been shown to contain triterpenes and **ergosterols**, which demonstrate broad antibiotic activity (Kandefer-Szerszen, 1982). Additionally, powerful purgative compounds contained in the fruiting body may have aided in addressing intestinal parasites known to have infected the Iceman (Stamets, 2002). Because the Birch Polypore was strung on a leather thong, others have pos-tulated that it had ornamental or ritual significance. The full answer may never be known, though few can dispute the significance of his carrying two common fungi that also have medicinal properties.

Mushrooms have been used for food, medicine, and ritual in a number of cultures for thousands of years. Our knowledge of the early history of traditional medicinal use is limited by a dearth of written material, and the relatively recent history of written records of any kind. In addition, our understanding of what species were used is based on the names by which fungi were known at the time, and the difficulty in translating those names into current taxonomy and nomenclature. For example, the mushroom the Greek physician Dioscordes referred to as Agaricon is now thought to be *Fomitopsis officinalis*, the Quinine Conk, but the names Agaricon and Agaric were also used for many other mushrooms.

The best records—and, indeed, the longest unbroken history of the use of mushrooms for medicine—come from the Chinese. Chinese culture and traditions are very fungi-phyllic, weaving mushrooms and other fungi into diet and health in ways few other cultures approach. History is written by the conquerors, reflecting their bias on the events and the times. Our understanding of the use of fungi in historic cultures has been limited by the ignorance and distrust of mushrooms on the part of the westerners who wrote accounts of their travels in other lands. Here is a brief review of some of the European, Asian, and Native American traditions of the medicinal use of fungi. (For a more in-depth look, refer to Hobbs, 1995.)

According to available records, Europeans used few medicinal mushrooms prior to the Renaissance. References were made to a mushroom, Agaricum, and its use as a moxa. In moxa, or moxibustion, the mushroom fruiting body or other herb was dried, shredded, and placed on the skin in an affected area. The material was then ignited and allowed to smolder on the skin to infuse the body with warmth and the mushroom's healing properties. This practice was used by Native Americans and is common in Traditional Chinese Medicine.

In the second century A.D., Dioscordes wrote an herbal treatise, *De Materia Medica,* which became the major reference work for healers in Europe for the next 1,700 years. Dioscordes held most mushrooms in ill favor, with the exception of Agaricon or the Agaric. Over time, the term *Agaricon* was applied to many woody polypores that grow on trees. Agaricon was looked upon as somewhat of a panacea and used to treat a number of illnesses, including diseases of the lungs, kidneys, spleen, and bladder, as well as fevers and pains. It was one ingredient in mithridate, a Roman herbal formula, and, much later, in Warburg's Tincture, a popular nineteenth-century formula (Hobbs, 1995). Warburg's Tincture was used to treat many ailments, chiefly tuberculosis and malaria, two scourges of the British Empire in the 1800s.

Beginning in the 1600s, mushrooms started to be more widely used in Europe. In addition to use as tonics (immune stimulators), several woody polypores and a number of dried Puffballs were employed as wound dressings and absorbents. Though some cultures, including the English, maintained a distrust of mushrooms and used them rarely for either food or medicine, other cultures made broad use of their fungal resources. In France, Italy, Poland, Russia, and other eastern European regions, mushrooms have long been a major part of the diet in addition to their medicinal use. Gathering and enjoying mushrooms is a family occupation and sport in many Baltic areas. As the Estonian saying goes: "Where there is a mushroom coming up, there is always a Russian waiting for it."

The native peoples of Russia and Poland have a long history of use of several medicinal mushrooms, including *Inonotus obliquus* (Chaga), a general tonic also used for intestinal disorders and many forms of cancer (Gorbunova et al., 2005). The Russians also used *Fomitopsis officinalis* (Quinine Conk) for many generations to heal numerous illnesses, and they began a centrally controlled study of its use in the beginning of the seventeenth century. *Amanita muscaria* (Fly Agaric) was historically used as both a sacred mushroom for communication with the divine and a general inebriant (Hobbs, 1995). *Fomes fomentarius*, known as Amadou in Europe, was used by peasants in Russia and surrounding countries as a styptic to stop bleeding and, later, as a treatment for indigestion and many forms of cancer. The same region used *Fomitopsis pinicola* (Red-belted Polypore) for its antitumor and sedative characteristics (Denisova, 2002). In the twentieth century, the use of Chaga led to a series of studies of its medicinal properties by the government of the U.S.S.R., culminating in the mid-1950s with the approval of a licensed medication made from Chaga and called Befungin. Befungin is still available in Russia, where it is used to treat a number of disorders.

The use of medicinal mushrooms by Native American tribes has varied greatly with the location of their home and their individual histories. Our knowledge of native medicinal practices from before the western colonization of North America is limited, overwhelmed by the dominant culture and the records of their use lost or discounted.

Traditional Chinese Medicine (TCM) and Mushrooms

The Chinese have recorded their use of mushrooms as medicine for at least 2,200 years, and it is thought by some that the knowledge contained in *De Materia*

Medica dates back 5,000 years (Smith et al., 2002). Much of the retained knowledge of medicinal practices in China can be attributed to the records of Taoist and Buddhist healers, as well as the long tradition of record-keeping by the Chinese government.

Traditional Chinese Medicine views the body as a system connected to nature and seeking to achieve and maintain balance in its world. Qi is life energy in circulation, and good health reflects a state where the qi is circulating through the body in a dynamic balance maintained by the interplay of the opposing energies of yin and yang.

Illness and its symptoms reflect an imbalance of energies leading to a state of disharmony. Viewed through the lens of TCM, disease indicates a need to restore harmony in our life energies through healthy living, including nutrition, exercise, and mental health. Interventions might include herbal remedies made up of or including medicinal mushrooms, or acupuncture, acupressure, and moxibustion, related practices that address the constriction of qi along body meridian lines. (Meridians are channels in our bodies in which qi circulates.)

A major difference between TCM and western medicine is TCM's focus on maintaining optimal health through a healthy lifestyle. *The goal is to support the body in order to promote the body's own self-healing potential.* Western medicine is often more focused on reacting to an illness once it has become a source of clinical significance in a person's life. Western medicine has made great strides in treating trauma, and there is no place I would rather be with a broken bone than in the United States under the care of a skilled trauma doctor. But after the physician has set the bone, stitched up the gash, or removed the offending tumor, it is up to the body to heal itself: knit the bone together, repair the skin and connective tissue, or coordinate the immune response to prevent infection. In order for the body to heal effectively, it must be in optimum condition, with reserves of energy, good nutrition, and a fully functioning immune system. Mushrooms or other health-promoting supplements serve as one aid to regaining or maintaining good health. Mushrooms are not a tool to use in isolation but are best used within the context of a healthy lifestyle.

Chapter 4

Our Immune System and How It Works

Our bodies are extremely complex living systems that have evolved over eons to be successful in an even more complex living world. Every day of our lives, our bodies are assaulted by other organisms seeking to use this warm, moist, nutrient-rich mass as a food source and living environment. Our skin, scalp, mouth, and digestive tract are home to millions of bacteria in a constantly shifting state of balance and generally living out their short lives without harm to us. Many of the bacteria that are benign or even beneficial residents in our bodies can become quite pathogenic if they get out of control. One example of this is the bacteria *Escherichia coli*, known by its more diminutive name, *E. coli*. Certain strains of *E. coli* are normal and prolific residents in the lower gastrointestinal tract, where they break down certain nutrients and, in the process, provide us with Vitamin K. Yet, *E. coli* growing in the gut cavity cause peritonitis and can quickly cripple or kill the victim. Others types of organisms, such as different species of bacteria, or even virulent strains of *E. coli*, viruses, and certain fungi, cause illness and even death. When we feel the symptoms of the flu, it is the end result of our body unsuccessfully fighting off the virus responsible for causing the flu. We are in constant contact with a panoply of microorganisms capable of causing illness, yet most of the time a healthy body prevents them from becoming established.

We also must contend with the fact that due to damage during DNA replication, or in response to harmful rays or chemicals, the body regularly produces malignant cells that, left unchecked, can grow rapidly to become cancer. It is the job of our immune system to detect and repel foreign invaders, as well as to respond to abnormal cells when they are detected. In a healthy body, this protective action happens many times each day, automatically and highly successfully. Cancerous tissue is stopped long before it becomes a problem, and infectious organisms are identified and destroyed before they can proliferate and trigger the symptoms of infection. Illness comes when our immune system is compromised and the infectious organism is able to set up housekeeping.

In even a healthy body, however, the immune system can become compromised by a number of factors. These can include poor nutrition, stress, an underlying illness or disorder, or that great American pastime "burning the candle at both ends." When we are exhausted, our entire system reflects our depletion, and we become an open door for illness.

The aging process is another cause of immune weakness. As we age, our immune system starts to lose strength, which is why the incidence of cancer increases markedly in middle and old age. Though we have made great strides toward understanding how the immune system functions, scientists readily concur that we have much to learn about this complex system on which so much of our health depends. So let's look at a basic primer on how the immune system functions, and in the next chapter I will address how mushrooms and fungal compounds can help support a functioning immune system. Keep in mind that this is a greatly simplified explanation. See the References section (page 132) for sources of more information.

Anthropomorphizing the Microbes

It is exceedingly difficult to discuss the immune system without using "us versus them" descriptions better suited to the battlefront journalist or historian than a mycologist. Try as I may, I find myself slipping back into the perception that infectious organisms and cancerous growths are like invasive armies seeking to storm the battlements and overwhelm the defenders. Though there is a part of me that clearly views germs as working-class organisms simply trying to make a place in the cell-eat-cell world in which we live, I cannot succeed in humanizing the little bugs. After all, I am one of the battlegrounds in which they live, and the degree of their success is in direct proportion to my own demise. So, you will see me slip into the non-objective reporting of the war correspondent while describing the workings of the immune system. I do not apologize that it comes across as self-serving. Charles Darwin, one of the earliest to focus our attention on the survival of the fittest, would certainly understand.

Elements of the Immune System

The immune system is a complex network of specialized tissues, cells, and chemicals, as well as the delivery system that takes them where they are needed. Basic defenses are concentrated where our vulnerable tissues are in constant contact with the outside world, including skin, mucous membranes, lungs, mouth, tear ducts, and the lining of the digestive tract. Bone marrow, spleen, tonsils, adenoids, lymph nodes, and the thymus gland all play major roles as sites of immune component production and concentration and are significant in immune defense.

Bone marrow is where basic white blood cells, or **lymphocytes**, evolve from precursor hematopoietic **stem cells**. The cells are then transported throughout the body using blood vessels or the lymphatic vessels, with major concentrations in the thymus, where **T-lymphocytes** (T-cells) mature, and in lymph nodes and other organs. Lymphocytes are major players in any immune response, and they mature into a number of very specialized cells, some of which we will examine more closely.

The lymphatic system communicates the presence of infection and inflammation and acts as a conduit for the elements of the immune response. The clear fluid carried by the lymphatic vessel network is called lymph. Composed of the interstitial fluid of cells and rich in various white blood cells, lymph is similar to blood plasma, with added white blood cells and a variety of chemical messengers.

The first requirement for an effective immune system is the body's ability to differentiate between self and non-self, and between healthy tissue and abnormal cells. In order to identify an invading organism, our body recognizes epitopes, protein markers on the outer surface of cells in the body. All of our own cells carry epitopes indicating their origin, and the immune response is directed only to those cells identified as foreign or malignant. This can be thought of as a recognition-and-response system: If the epitopes are seen as "foreign," the body triggers a response to isolate the invaders and eliminate them through lysis (cell destruction) or, in some cases, through phagocytosis (engulfment and digestion) by large lymphocytes called **macrophages**.

Any foreign body capable of triggering an immune response is called an **antigen**. Antigens can include whole cells, or fragments of bacteria or virus and a host of other particles or cells. The cells from another person, also antigens, trigger an immune response that forms the basis of tissue rejection following a transplant of blood, tissue, or organs. Many, but not all, common antigens are proteins, but they can also be other particles. It is thought that the complex polysaccharides produced in mushrooms, such as glucans, present themselves to immune cells in such a manner that they trigger an antigen response.

When a normal cell becomes malignant or cancerous, some of the protein markers on its surface change, and the immune system identifies the cell as foreign and takes steps to eliminate it. A problem with certain cancer types, and with tumors that have become well established, is that they develop the ability to hide from an immune response.

Our immune system can be divided into two main branches, **innate immunity** and **acquired immunity**.

The Innate Immune System

The innate immune system encompasses the basic elements of resistance present at birth or developed very early in life. It includes the physical and chemical barrier of the skin; the sticky trapping fluid of mucous membranes; the antibacterial chemicals in tears, sweat, and nasal secretions; and the acidic and protein-digesting enzymes in the stomach. In addition, the mechanical action of cilia removing debris from the lungs, the expulsory action of coughing and sneezing, and the flushing action of tears, saliva, and urine all act as barriers to infection. Another innate immune response is the physiologic actions of elevated temperature, pH changes (e.g., in the stomach), and oxygen tension.

The innate immune system also comprises white blood cells such as **natural killer** (NK) cells, **dendritic cells** (DCs), and macrophages. These are designed to recognize and destroy foreign cells and, at times, to trigger a broader immune response as a result of encountering antigens. This more coordinated response happens when a macrophage, encountering a bacteria or other antigen, engulfs it, breaks it into antigen bits, and transports these bits of protein to a **B-cell**. It is a nonspecific response, meaning that the macrophage is not actively seeking out that specific bacteria but is able to respond to a wide range of antigens coming into contact with it.

Natural killer cells are vital lymphocytes, which make up to 15 percent of the body's white blood cells. They are charged with holding the front line in the initial defense against invasive bacteria, viruses, and malignant cells. Circulating throughout the body, NK cells respond to certain protein markers on foreign cell surfaces and destroy the cells; they also recognize cells lacking self-identification molecules. Thus NK cells have the potential to attack many types of foreign cells.

Dendritic cells, sometimes called Langerhans cells, are immune cells that start out in an immature stage in the bone marrow. They then become part of the surface of a number of tissues in high contact with the outside world where innate immune response is needed. These include the skin, lungs, stomach, and intestine, where DCs develop asymmetrically to present as much surface area as possible to foreign particles entering the body. These immature DCs sample passing cells and particles, and when they encounter antigens, they take action by maturing and carrying the fragments of antigen to the nearest lymph tissue or to the spleen, where they are presented to T-cells. Known as one of several antigen-presenting cells, DCs then help activate the T-cells as they prepare a specific response to the antigen.

An additional important component of innate immunity are the **phagocytic cells,** including macrophages, which do not require activation but can destroy certain infected or abnormal cells. Macrophages develop from **monocytes**, immature phagocytic cells circulating in the blood, and are found in highest concentrations in organs such as the lungs, liver, and kidneys, where they act as scavengers to remove aging or worn-out cells. They also produce and release a variety of chemical messengers and effectors, including **tumor necrosis factor** (TNF), an important component in inflammation response.

NK cells and macrophages also release cytokines that activate elements in the acquired immune system, notably B- and T-cells, as a second line of defense. Neutrophils, another type of phagocyte, are filled with granules of potent chemicals that, when injected into a harmful cell or bacteria, break down and destroy the cell.

The Acquired Immune System

The acquired immune system, as the name implies, develops over time in response to invading organisms. The body develops acquired immunity in response to an early threat from a particular invasive organism, such as a specific type of bacteria. The acquired immune response requires a functioning immune system. The need for a functioning immune system will become very important when we examine how fungal glucans and other polysaccharides work within the body.

The foundation of the acquired immune response is the action of T-cells and B-cells to produce **antibodies** in response to a new antigen. These antibodies are specific to the antigen that triggered their production and help eliminate that type of antigen or cells containing that antigen. Human antibodies belong to a class of large proteins called immunoglobulins. We lack antibodies at birth because the newborn has not yet been exposed to antigens that trigger their production, though some initial antibody protection can be conferred through a mother's milk. That alone is a strong argument for breast-feeding your newborn.

B-cell and T-cell lymphocytes are types of specialized white blood cells. T-cells, matured from white blood cells in the thymus, can directly destroy invasive cells and also regulate a broader attack on an infection by calling in other immune cells and triggering their activity. In this triggering role they are known as helper T-cells. Cytotoxic (killer) T-cells have the major responsibility of destroying our own cells when they become infected or cancerous. This function also results in tissue rejection following a transplant.

B-cells are major players in the production of antibodies. A macrophage or dendritic cell from the innate immune system captures and transports a specific antigen to a B-cell. The B-cell, with the assistance of a helper T-cell, matures into a **plasma cell** and makes antibodies, up to 10 million an hour, to attack the specific antigen. The antibodies are then circulated throughout the body to locate any presenting antigens (read bacteria or virus), marking the cell for destruction by a macrophage or by the complement system. The complement system is a series of proteins that act in concert to destroy antibody-marked invasive cells. The sequence that results in the death of the invasive cell by complement is called **apoptosis,** or **programmed cell death.**

After an initial immune response—for example, after you overcome a viral infection—some of the antibodies produced to fight the infection continue to circulate within specialized B-cells called **memory cells**. If the same antigen enters the body again, the memory cell quickly recognizes it and addresses the attack by becoming a plasma cell and producing antibodies. Memory cells continue to be active in the body for many years after being formed and are the basis of vaccination immunity effectiveness. When I get a flu vaccine in the early winter, I am being injected with antigens to the strains of flu virus most active that year. My immune system responds by producing antibodies to that specific strain. Some of those antibodies are stored in memory cells, so if I come into contact with the virus at a later date, those memory cells will rapidly flood my system with antibodies to fight off the virus. Thus I say I am "immune" to that strain of the flu. Of course, the nimble flu virus is busy mutating into a slightly different strain capable of bypassing the current antibody.

Both B-cells and T-cells produce cytokines to alert the body to the need for an immune response. Some cytokines also act to inhibit viral replication **(interferons)** or activate macrophages (TNF), and can directly attack and kill cancer and other invasive cells. Cytokines are small proteins with several functions, including relating messages, triggering responses, working in concert with other cells to either promote or inhibit a particular action, and acting directly, as cytotoxic molecules, against foreign cells.

When normal cells in the body become malignant, as in the case of cancer cells, the nature of the antigens on their cell surface changes. Like any other cell, these cells will shed some of these bits of protein that mark them and, as tumor antigens, enter the circulatory system. The presence of the tumor antigen is noted by macrophages and T-cells, which remove the antigen bits and trigger a more coordinated response to destroy the cancerous cells. A tumor will continue to grow in situations where the immune system's search-and-destroy function breaks down.

Many of the same factors that make us more vulnerable to infection also add to our vulnerability to cancer growth. These include factors outside our control such as environmental toxins and aging, as well as those factors more often within our control such as stress, nutrition, level of exhaustion, etc.

Our immune system, composed of overlapping and redundant components, is remarkable in both its complexity and its ability to defend us from the pathogens entering the body as well as the malignant or damaged cells of our body. It is able to perform this remarkable job without damage to the healthy tissue of the body. It is important to understand the basic functioning of the immune system in order to explore the action of medicinal mushrooms in supporting and strengthening immunity. Though this review may seem quite complex, it represents a significant simplification of the immune system. For more information and a treatment in greater depth, please refer to the NIH publication that is one source of my information: *Understanding the Immune System: How It Works,* available at http://www.niaid.nih.gov/Publications/immune/the_immune_system.pdf www3.niaid.nih.gov/topics/immuneTolerance/

Chapter 5

The Medicinal Components of Mushrooms

In 1776, when the American colonies declared their independence, the average life expectancy was around thirty-seven years. By 1900, our average life expectancy had increased to about forty-nine years, and in this new millennium Americans are expected to live well into their mid-seventies on average. The main reason for this increasing longevity is our success in battling infectious disease and the corresponding decrease in infant mortality.

Antibiotics have been the major contributor to the mix, and we can thank fungi for that. Where a few generations ago a sickly child might not have survived to attend school, our medical skill and our understanding of infectious processes and antibiotic treatment now generally ensure that even a child with poor health will survive to adulthood. Until very recently in our evolution, few humans lived past the age of fifty. We now know that the human immune system and other bodily systems begin to decline as we age. Cancer, an illness that markedly increases with age as well as in response to toxins, was not common or well recognized until the twentieth century. I recently noted a statistic stating that two of five people have experienced cancer by age sixty-five. After age fifty, our immune system is coping with a body in early senescence and can use all the support and care we can provide.

We live in a time with an astoundingly high degree of daily stress. America is known throughout Europe for a slavish work ethic and a reluctance to use the relatively few days of vacation bestowed upon us. We work longer hours to compete in the workplace and feel less secure that our jobs will be here next year. We are living in the midst of a crowded, noisy, intrusive, complex, and conflict-ridden world where most of us remain closely attuned to the negative headlines and fear-based media missives. "Having it all" comes with the high price of increased stress, as the definition of "enough" seems to be as constantly expanding as the big-bang universe. Increasingly the food we eat is more highly processed, resulting in a loss of many of the nutrients contained in fresh food. We face these exponentially changing societal and cultural trends living in bodies that evolve at a much slower pace than our culture has.

When our immune system is compromised and our body and psyche are under stress, we are more vulnerable to opportunistic infections such as the common cold or flu. We can all hear the maternal voice in our head telling us, "If you don't take care of yourself, you'll get sick." Of course, all those voices, internal and external, telling us to practice good self-care are right. Not only are we more vulnerable to infection from viruses, fungi, or bacteria, but our body is also less able to monitor and reject cells that have become cancerous when our immune system is compromised by poor nutrition, increasing age, and stress.

In our normal functioning, our body regularly makes malignant or potentially cancerous cells. This occurs as a result of mistakes in cell replication, or it can be triggered by radiation, toxins, or other external forces. Changes in the cell wall proteins of malignant cells enable immune system dendritic cells, macrophages, and T-cells to recognize the "bad" cell, and to destroy it or target it and others like it for removal.

Remember, recognition of self and non-self, including malignant or damaged self-cells, is a cornerstone of our immune system. An immune system compromised by age, stress, poor nutrition, or other factors is less efficient at keeping up with the need to clear malignant cells from the body. In addition, some tumors can hide from our immune system, enabling the cancer to proliferate before it is detected.

Good nutrition, lowered stress, and an otherwise healthy lifestyle are vitally important to keep the body and immune system functioning optimally. We can also take steps to actively support the immune system. **Immunotherapy** utilizing one or a combination of immune system stimulants is becoming increasingly common as one tool for addressing a number of conditions, including cancer, opportunistic infections, and other systemic concerns.

Mushrooms have been used as medicine for thousands of years in many cultures, especially in China, Japan, and parts of eastern and northern Europe. Many are recognized as a traditional tonic, something that stimulates the physical or mental vigor of the recipient. Medicinal mushrooms are known for giving our immune system a kick-start and increasing the healing potential of the body. Someone whose immune system is somewhat stimulated is generally considered more protected from infection and better able to dispose of unhealthy cells.

Compounds found in many mushrooms can modulate the functioning of our immune system. Though some mushroom components are able to directly attack microbes or tumor cells in the body, most fungal medicinal compounds are considered **immunoceuticals** rather than drugs. Their effectiveness comes from working with the immune system to function with increased vigor rather than having a direct **cytotoxic** effect on cancer or infection. This is an important distinction for a number of reasons. Mushroom polysaccharides work with a functioning immune system to increase its activity and effectiveness, and a more efficient immune response can help the body ward off the many opportunistic infections that lurk in our daily lives as well as remove malignant cells.

Western medicine has made great strides in understanding the causes of major infectious diseases and, in the case of those caused by bacteria or viruses, developing antibiotics to combat the infections. We have also become very adept at treating the body after trauma. Both these cases involve an assault on the body and addressing the symptoms of the assault after the system has become compromised.

Our bodies themselves, however, have enormous potential for healing injury and fighting infection, and it is very important that we learn to support them in this work. Western medicine, by and large, has not followed the lead of eastern health practitioners, who focus on diagnosing the healing capacity of the body and intervening to support the optimal functioning of that healing system. The Chinese call it qi, or chi, the Japanese ki, and it is the embodiment of life force—literally the air, breath, or force of life. A basic goal of Traditional Chinese Medicine is to establish and maintain the optimal flow of qi in the body. Another way this is often conceptualized is to seek to maintain or re-establish a balance in the bodily and spiritual systems.

There has been an increase in alternative health practitioners in this country who focus on the living system holistically and seek to address the weaknesses of the bodily systems in order to support health. Many western-trained medical doctors are integrating a more holistic focus on the body-mind-spirit connection into their practice. Concerned people turn to good diet and healthy lifestyle first and the use of supplemental interventions, including natural products such as herbs, nutrition, and nutritional supplements and functional foods, as part of their effort to support the body's natural immune response. For generations, eastern practitioners have recognized the effectiveness of medicinal mushrooms and specific herbs as nutritional supplements to improve the functioning of specific organs and bodily systems. We have called them tonics, immune boosters, immune support, immunoceuticals, and similar names.

Mushroom Polysaccharides and Health

The cell walls of mushrooms contain long chains of complex sugars called polysaccharides (literally translated as "many sugars"). The polysaccharides are significant structural components of the cells, giving them a rigid strength. Some of these diverse polysaccharides have been shown to act within a mammalian system to stimulate the functioning of some components of the immune system. To date, more than 650 species of mushrooms, representing in excess of 180 genera, have been shown to possess immune stimulating and antitumor polysaccharides (Fan et al., 2006). Within this group, few mushroom species have undergone more than the simple screening of the biologic activity of a crude polysaccharide extract. The polysaccharides that have been examined take an astounding variety of forms with a complex variety of side branching, helical configurations, attached proteins, acid groups, and other variations. The innumerable forms these polysaccharides take determine the compounds they form and their specific action within the living system of those who eat them. In plants, the major polysaccharide molecules making up cell walls are cellulose and related compounds. In fungi cell walls, they are predominantly chitins and glucans.

Glucans: Glucans are polysaccharides of high to very high molecular weight, constructed of units of glucose and containing variously branched side chains. Found in a number of different species of plants and fungi, glucans serve as structural building blocks to make cell walls rigid. Some mushrooms contain more than 30 percent glucans by dry weight, especially those mushrooms with a dense, woody texture, such as Artist's Conk.

Glucans exist in an incredible variety of size and configuration as reflected in their range of biologic activity. Some branching patterns of glucans have been shown to have a significant positive impact on their biologic action. Though glucans with beta-1,3 and beta-1,6 branching appear to be the most active in stimulating immune response, other branching patterns in polysaccharides are effective in immune modulation (Lindequist et al., 2005). In general, increases in size and complexity of branching correspond with increased biologic activity (Ohno, 2005).

There are also exceptions to this rule. Some researchers acknowledge that using a mixture of mushroom species with a wide variation of glucans is likely to trigger a broader-based immune response (Stamets, 2000). For this reason we are seeing more nutraceuticals on the market composed of multiple species of mushrooms. Some mushrooms contain glucans as well as structural polysaccharides made up of sugar units other than glucose. These also can stimulate immune response.

Glucans are not readily available without first cooking the mushroom to break down the structure of the cell walls. Almost all wild edible mushrooms must be cooked before eating to increase their digestibility. Some cases of mushroom "poisoning" are due to people eating uncooked or undercooked mushrooms and becoming ill due to the indigestibility of their meal or the presence of a toxin that would have been neutralized by the heat of cooking. Morels, for instance, will sicken the person who eats them raw. With mushrooms used for medicinal purposes, the need for cooking is doubly true: Cooking makes the mushrooms digestible as food and also helps release the active polysaccharides that would otherwise remain bound up in the indigestible cell wall structure.

Some beta glucans are too large to be absorbed through the gut and into our bodies. An example of this is the proprietary medicinal compound Lentinan, isolated from Shiitake. Often delivered by injection into the peritoneal cavity, it was thought to be ineffective if taken by mouth. More recent research has shown that Lentinan taken orally triggers the same response as when injected, though it takes a higher oral dose to get the same level of immune response (Ohno, 2005). Though Lentinan does not seem to be absorbed through the gut, the glucans triggers an immune response nonetheless by acting on the immune effector cells in the digestive mucosa lining the gut and intestines and in the tonsils and adenoids. Undigested glucans and other structural components of mushrooms, such as chitin, are passed out of the gastrointestinal tract as fiber. This is why a diet rich in mushrooms can help ensure bowel regularity or, in some people accustomed to a low-fiber diet, act as a laxative.

Mushroom polysaccharides taken orally or injected into the stomach cavity can stimulate the immune system in a number of ways, depending on their configuration. Glucans, because they are not naturally found in animals, are considered to be classic pattern-recognition molecules when encountered in the body by elements of the innate immune system such as natural killer cells (Takeda and Okumura, 2004). In other words, the body views them as a possible invading organism and acts to protect itself. The site of recognition seems to be surface receptors on immune cells such as NK cells or macrophages. which then secrete small proteins that induce programmed cell death, known as apoptosis. Both NK cells and macrophages also release certain messenger cytokines to activate effector cells such as T-cells and other macrophages and NK cells. The activating cytokines include certain forms of TNF, interferons, and interleukins, and the stimulation of all these immune cells results in more potential for the body to respond to invasive organisms and tumor cells.

The specific modes of action of glucans are summarized in the table at right. Please refer to the chapters on specific mushroom species for more information.

Mushroom Polysaccharides and Their Effects	
Immune System Component	**Effects of Medicinal Mushroom Polysaccharides**
Natural Killer Cells (NK cells) (Takeda, 2004)	Structure of polysaccharide directly stimulates activity of NK cells to: <ul><li>Lysis of invasive or malignant cells directly.</li><li>Release messenger proteins such as interleukins to signal and activate other immune cells such as macrophages and T-cells.</li><li>Release interferon-gamma to suppress viral replication and proliferation.</li><li>Release tumor necrosis factor-alpha to induce apoptotic cell death in target cells.</li></ul>
Macrophages	<ul><li>Activation of macrophages for increased anti-microbial activity and increased scavenging activity.</li><li>Production and secretion of tumor necrosis factor alpha.</li><li>Production and secretion of several interleukins responsible for signaling or stimulating other immune cells into action, including T-Cells, B-Cells, NK cells, mast cells, and plasma cells.</li></ul>
T-Cells	Induced maturation of T-helper cells and favors the maturation of T-H1 over T-H2 cells, which favors enhanced cellular immunity. <ul><li>T-helper cells are active in the maturation of B-cells, which in turn trigger the maturation and action of directly Cytotoxic T-cells.</li><li>T-helper cells activate macrophages.</li></ul>
B-Cells	Certain polysaccharides directly stimulate B-Cell activation and production of antibody to tumor antigen and other antigens. Other polysaccharides have been shown to reduce antibody production.

Complement	Some mushroom polysaccharides have been shown to stimulate production and/or activation of C-3, a key component in the complement system and responsible for setting up antibacterial response in the complement system.
Tumor Necrosis Factor, or TNF-alpha	Most bioactive mushroom polysaccharides have been shown to stimulate macrophages resulting in increased release of TNF-alpha, responsible for: • Induction of apoptotic cell death in targeted tumor or microbe cells. • Induction of inflammatory reaction. • Stimulation of phagocytosis.
Interleukins (IL)	Application of polysaccharides from a range of species has been shown to increase the concentration of a number of interleukins responsible for triggering the maturation of other immune cells and coordinating immune responses. Some of the interleukins involved include IL-1, IL-2, IL-8, IL-12, IL-6, and IL-10.
Interferons	A number of polysaccharides from mushrooms have been shown to trigger an increased production of Interferon alpha (Inf-alpha) from white blood cells. Inf-alpha is responsible for viral resistance in the body.
Dendritic Cells (DCs)	Several mushroom extracts have been shown to trigger increased endocytic activity, maturation of immature DCs and to trigger DCs in their role of maturation of naïve T-cells (Lull et al, 2005).

Proteoglycans: A proteoglycan is a large molecule made up of a polysaccharide or a mixture of polysaccharides linked to the amino acids of a protein. In Turkey Tail mushrooms, the proteoglycan PSK is made up primarily of glucose units and a smaller percentage of other simple sugars in a classic branched glucan pattern and linked to proteins. In a proteoglycan, it is the polysaccharide branches, similar to glucans, that trigger immune response.

Studies indicate that the glucan component is responsible for the activation of innate and adaptive immune response in normal, healthy subjects as well as those coping with cancers (Kato et al., 1995). It has been repeatedly shown that PSK, other proteoglycans, and the glucans alone act to stimulate a functioning immune system, so it is important to begin their use before engaging in treatment that compromises immune functioning. This would include chemotherapy or radiation, treatments that can temporarily depress or shut down aspects of the immune system. If you face this situation, please discuss it with your health care provider.

Ergosterol: This substance is to fungi what cholesterols are to mammals. In fungi, ergosterol is a component of cell walls and may be important in regulating the permeability of the membranes, thereby regulating the flow of water and molecules into and out of the cells. Ergosterol is a lipid in the form of sterol, and a precursor or provitamin to Vitamin D2. In the presence of sunlight (or artificial ultraviolet light), ergosterol is converted to Vitamin D. Vitamin D is increasingly heralded for its role in the prevention of cancers by increasing immune system phagocytosis (the engulfing and destroying) of cancer cells, and facilitation of other **immunomodulatory** functions. In addition, it is responsible for regulation and absorption of calcium and phosphorus and thus important in promoting optimal bone growth and preventing osteoporosis.

Terpenes, including diterpenes, triterpenes, and sesquiterpenes: Terpenes are likely the most numerous of organic compounds, with at least 23,000 already described and more being discovered daily (Wang et al., 2005). They are primarily formed and used by plants and fungi but are also found to a smaller extent in animals. Triterpenes are often precursors to steroids in both plants and animals and to other hormones in animals. Given the vast number and variation within this group, it is not surprising to find that the range of function within the terpenes is equally vast. As secondary chemicals, they protect the fungus from a host of predators ranging from bacteria and other fungi to hungry humans. Terpenes are implicated in many of the gastrointestinal poisonings caused by some species of mushrooms.

Terpenes' role as medicinal components manufactured by fungi include direct cytotoxic action against tumor cells and direct antibacterial, antifungal, and antiviral effects. Various terpenes have also been shown to have significant **antioxidant** capabilities. Another area of promising research has led to the use of some medicinal mushrooms for the production of anti-inflammatory compounds. A number of terpenes from mushrooms have been shown to block some of the key pathways to an inflammatory response (Von Kemami Wangun, 2006), and these mushrooms, including Reishi, Chaga, and a few other polypores, are being used informally for their anti-inflammatory effects.

Vitamins: Most mushrooms contain significant amounts of several water-soluble vitamins, including Vitamin C and the B vitamins niacin, riboflavin, and pantothenic acid. Some mushrooms also contain amounts of Vitamin E and K, and Vitamin D, as mentioned above.

In a recent fascinating discovery, mushrooms exposed to ultraviolet light before or after harvest quickly converted the ergosterol to vitamin D2 in astounding amounts. In *Mycelium Running* (pp. 202–4), Paul Stamets reported several experiments where the levels of Vitamin D were increased by more than a hundred times for mushrooms dried in sunlight as compared to those dried in the dark. This happens with both Maitake and Shiitake. The increase was such that anyone indiscriminately eating sun-dried mushrooms could easily get an overdose, though I have found no reported incidences of Vitamin D toxicity with mushrooms.

An Aside on the Role of Reductionist Tendencies (and Money) in the Formulation of Mushroom Medicines

If you examine the scientific research on medicinal mushrooms conducted over the past forty years, you will note that most of the studies that have moved beyond basic evaluations have focused on a handful of species: Turkey Tail, Maitake, Shiitake, Reishi, and *Schizophyllum*. Recently the top five have been joined by *Agaricus blazii,* Oysters, *Phellinus lentius,* Comb Tooth, and, to a lesser extent, Chaga. Most of these species have a long history of use in traditional medicine and have shown clear evidence of healing properties. In addition—and perhaps as important in the ways of the world and the role of Big Pharma in medicine—most of these species have one or more licensed "proprietary" compounds. A proprietary compound is one that has been isolated, named, and licensed and is now used in clinical trials to test for effectiveness as medicine. The "proprietor" controls access to and use of the compound, and reaps profits from others' use of it. Proprietary compounds are usually marketed under their trade name.

Crude extracts of mushrooms make it more difficult to draw conclusions about cause and effect. Medical practitioners and researchers around the world have been calling for isolated **fractions** in order to be more confident about the purity of the compounds, as well as the predictability of the substances, especially in clinical situations with human subjects. Other vital issues needing resolution on the path toward approval of fungi as a "medicine" in western medicine include:

- Appropriate dosage in clinical applications
- Safety of use in clinical settings
- Side effects
- Interactions with other medications, foods, etc.
- Effects of extended use on a broad range of human subjects

There are significant costs associated with the process needed to have a promising substance approved as a medicine in the United States. In a brief article in *Psychiatry News,* Mark Moran (2003) reported that by the late 1990s the average cost of bringing a new medication through the research and development phase in the United States was $897 million, and we can be sure that the cost is now in the billions of dollars. The process also takes time, between ten and fifteen years from development to approval and finally to market in the United States. For this reason, few nonproprietary compounds are supported through the approval process, since their profit would not accrue to one company. This may be why more of the mushroom products sold as dietary supplements consist of either a single mushroom or mixed mushroom compounds. The positive benefits to this are the ready availability of these potentially helpful supplements. The downside includes, in some cases, a lack of clinical research involving human subjects; less information regarding purity and appropriate dosage; and reduced confidence in the usefulness of the products.

In Japan, the second most widely used medication used to treat cancer is an isolated proprietary compound of Turkey Tail. Called PSK and marketed as Krestin, it is responsible for several hundred million dollars in sales annually in Asia (Stamets, 2000). In the United States, PSK is in phase II clinical trials for approval for use in cancer treatment. Though PSK is marketed as a purified extract of the mushroom, in reality it contains a mix of polysaccharides and proteanated polysaccharides.

As mentioned earlier, there is increasing evidence that the most broad-based and arguably effective stimulation of the immune system may result from the action of an array of mushroom polysaccharides. The trend toward isolating one compound for use as a drug may dilute the potential positive impact on the individual in need. Clearly, it will not dilute the bottom line of the pharmaceutical company that holds the license to produce the compound, though it will help recover the research and development costs.

Chapter 6

Mushrooms as Functional Food

Beginning in the 1990s, nutritionists focusing on the evils of fat touted mushrooms as a healthy alternative to meat. Mushrooms were valued for what they did not have: fat, cholesterol, and calories. With the increasing recognition that some mushrooms have medicinal value in addition to being tasty, low-calorie plate-fillers, we need to redefine our view of fungi as food.

Mushrooms once were seen as a nutrient vacuum, having flavor and texture but little nutritional value. Today we know this is not true. Beyond their excellent and varied taste, mushrooms represent a good source of crude protein as well as several needed vitamins. Most edible mushrooms contain from 1 to 4 percent fresh weight and 19 to 40 percent dry weight protein, generally with a good complement of amino acids, though lowest in a couple of sulfur-containing amino acids. Mushrooms rank below fresh meat and above milk and almost all vegetables as a source of dietary protein (Chang and Miles, 2004). They possess useful amounts of Vitamins B1, B2, and C, niacin, and biotin. They also contain relatively high amounts of ergosterol, or Provitamin D2, and are a good source of this essential precursor to Vitamin D. The essential minerals potassium, sodium, phosphorus, magnesium, and calcium are found in mushrooms. They also provide the trace minerals copper, zinc, iron, manganese, molybdenum, cadmium, and selenium. Mushrooms also have relatively high amounts of indigestible carbohydrates in the form of crude fiber.

Because they are high in water content and low in both fats and indigestible carbohydrates, mushrooms eaten alone are not a great source of burnable energy. Many of the flavor elements of mushrooms are soluble by fats; perhaps that is why we have learned to sauté them in butter or olive oil.

Mushrooms are valued for their nutritional content, but this does not explain why some species are recommended as a dietary supplement, **nutraceutical**, or **functional food**. It is the structure of their glucans and related polysaccharides, along with the presence of secondary chemical compounds, including terpenes, that makes them important as functional food beyond good nutrition. As a functional food, mushrooms cannot be said to cure disease, as this has not been established to the satisfaction of the U.S. government's Federal Food and Drug

Administration (FDA). A mushroom nutraceutical has been defined as a fruiting body, or mycelium extract, from a mushroom or mixture of mushrooms consumed not as food but as capsules, powders, or liquid extracts and having a potentially therapeutic application (Chang and Buswell, 1996). The value of mushroom nutraceuticals worldwide grew from an estimated $3.8 billion in 1994 to more than $6 billion in 2000, with North American sales contributing less than 1 percent. Demand in the United States has grown an estimated 20 to 40 percent annually, depending on the mushroom species (Chang and Miles, 2004), and represents great potential for the future.

There is a difference between consuming mushroom extracts and products as a form of therapy and eating health-promoting mushrooms as a part of a healthy diet. In the words of the Greek physician Hippocrates in the fifth century B.C., "Let food be your medicine and medicine be your food," a philosophy to which we find ourselves returning following a too-long experiment with the industrial food complex. From our growing awareness of the interrelationships among diet, health, and disease, we have spawned the concept of functional food as a way to talk about those foods particularly useful in health maintenance. Though a consensus definition of functional food is yet to come, it is generally accepted to mean foods intended to be consumed as part of the normal diet and containing biologically active components that offer the potential of enhanced health or reduced risk of disease. At times, the term also encompasses some processed food products or extracts, though this may be due more to lobbying by food processors unwilling to miss out on the positive association of health-promoting food.

Functional-food science and the increasingly clear recommendations regarding the components of a healthy diet come from a growing understanding of the negative impact of eating large, calorie-rich meals composed of processed, high-fat, and high-carbohydrate, but nutrient-deficient, ingredients. This style of eating has led Americans—and, increasingly, other populations throughout the world—into an epidemic of obesity, type 2 diabetes, high blood pressure, and a host of associated diet- and exercise-related disorders. The opposite is also true, as shown in the growing understanding of the benefits of a healthy, balanced diet and regular activity in maintaining and reclaiming optimum health.

We are what we eat, and if the diet is heavy in Twinkies, by the time a Twinkie-lover reaches middle age, there is a good chance he or she will begin to resemble one. On the other hand, we also have learned how many lifestyle-related diseases can be reversed through healthy diet and exercise practices. Even the lungs of a smoker, despite having been polluted by smoke for many years, can repair much of the damage if a person stops smoking.

Due to all their nutritional value and the potential health-promoting benefits of medicinal species, mushrooms are a great example of a functional food worth incorporating in your diet. To date, I know of only one study that looks at the health outcomes related to regular consumption of a medicinal mushroom in a large population. Health officials in the Nagano prefecture of Japan noted that the region had a lower incidence of stomach cancers when compared to adjacent prefectures and to Japan as a whole. A study from 1972 to 1986 revealed that mushroom farmers in the area had a lower death rate from cancer than others, and the consumption of mushrooms was suggested as the protective factor (Ikekawa, 2005). Further case studies between 1998 and 2002 showed a relationship between the frequency of eating three species of edible and medicinal mushrooms and the rates of stomach cancer in the same region. Those individuals consuming mushrooms at least once a week had a lower incidence of cancers. The mushrooms were *Flammulina velutipes, Pholiota namelo,* and *Hypsizygus marmoreus.* Of the three, only *Flammulina* occurs naturally in New England. These studies suggest that the regular consumption of medicinal mushrooms as food can have a cancer-deterrent effect.

Over time, developing a stable supply of medicinal mushrooms and preserving them for use throughout the year is one way to increase regular intake of healthy functional food. For me, the process of exploration, collecting, and identifying mushrooms is also a beneficial practice. I often use the time as a walking meditation, tuned into the natural environment and strolling with no more important goal than looking for good oaks, hemlocks, and other habitat trees. Using your spare time in September and October to scout areas with mature oak trees will likely reveal a few productive Maitake trees. Just a couple of such trees can provide you with many pounds of edible medicinal mushrooms for table and freezer.

It is also relatively easy to prepare simple tinctures and powders of fruiting bodies to support health during stressful periods throughout the year. In the winter, for instance, I start my day with a mixed medicinal mushroom tincture (Immune Blend), with Chaga added, as a way to support my constitutionally weak respiratory system. Before I increased my use of medicinal mushrooms five years ago, I suffered from at least one, and often more, bouts of bronchitis each winter and spring. I have not had bronchitis in five years.

Medicinal Mushroom Species

Northeastern Medicinal Mushrooms and Their Uses

Common Name	Species Name	Antitumor/ Immune-stimulating	Immunomodulator	Anti-inflammatory	Liver tonic/ Liver protection	Cholesterol/ Lipid regulation	Antibacterial	Antiviral	Pain relief	Kidney tonic	Antioxidant	Cardiovascular/ Blood pressure	Lungs/Respiratory	Nerve tonic
Tinder Conk, Amadou	*Fomes fomentarius*	✓					✓	✓						
Red-belted Polypore	*Fomitopsis pinicola*	✓		✓	✓		✓							
Artist's Conk	*Ganoderma applanatum*	✓	✓	✓			✓	✓					✓	
Varnish Conk, Reishi	*Ganoderma lucidum, G. tsugae*	✓	✓	✓	✓	✓	✓	✓	✓			✓	✓	✓
Maitake, Hen of the Woods	*Grifola frondosa*	✓	✓		✓		✓	✓				✓		
Comb Tooth, Lion's Mane, Bear's Head Tooth	*Hericium americanum, H. coralloides*	✓	✓				✓						✓	✓
Chaga, Birch Clinker	*Inonotus obliquus*	✓	✓	✓	✓		✓		✓				✓	
Birch Polypore	*Piptoporus betulinus*	✓					✓							
Oyster Mushroom	*Pleurotus ostreatus, P. populinus*	✓				✓	✓	✓						
Turkey Tail	*Trametes versicolor*	✓	✓				✓	✓		✓				
Other Medicinal Mushrooms Not Covered in Detail in This Book														
Honey Mushroom	*Armillaria mellea complex*											✓		
Umbrella Polypore	*Polyporus umbellatus*	✓	✓	✓	✓		✓	✓		✓	✓		✓	
Shiitake	*Lentinula edodes*	✓	✓		✓	✓	✓	✓		✓		✓		
Split Gill	*Schizophyllum commune*	✓	✓	✓	✓		✓			✓				
False Tinder Conk	*Phellinus igniarius*	✓	✓											

Chapter 7

Reishi *(Ganoderma tsugae* and *G. lucidum)*

Common names: Hemlock Varnished Conk, Varnished Conk; Reishi (Japan); Ling Zhi (China); Hemlock Polypore, Red Reishi (PHOTOGRAPHS ON PAGES 65–67)

Of the myriad aspects of mushrooms that fascinate me, one of the first and most enduring is their incredible beauty and grace of form. My first encounters with the diversity of fungi occurred in the deeply verdant forests and fields of upstate New York in the early 1970s. Fresh from the deserts of New Mexico, I was captivated by the color, form, and delicate beauty of the many mushrooms I saw.

Few species of mushrooms can match the heart-stopping beauty of the Varnished Conks. Growing on hardwoods or hemlock, these close species are stunning in their presentation of lacquered, dark-red hues blending into the growing edges of yellows and whites. Their varied growth forms, jutting off the side or the top of wood, are equally impressive. Coming upon a hemlock with a trunk two feet in diameter festooned with numerous Reishi mushrooms like so many dark-red glistening jewels is a deeply awe-inspiring sight. Their beauty is matched only by their status as a medicinal mushroom of the highest repute. The Chinese call *G. lucidum* Mushroom of Immortality and Herb of Spiritual Potency (Hobbs, 1995), references to the respect they have for these mushrooms.

A Note on Species Distinction within the Genus *Ganoderma*

There are primarily two species of varnished-cap *Ganoderma* in the Northeast: *G. tsugae*, found growing on hemlock throughout the region, and *G. lucidum,* found growing on hardwood deciduous trees from southern New England to the tropics. A third, *G. curtisii*, grows from Massachusetts south into the southeastern United States and west to Nebraska. It also inhabits hardwoods and is generally distinguished by its more yellow-ochre color tones.

Many mushroom taxonomists do not distinguish *G. curtisii* from *G. lucidum* (Kuo, 2004, and Volk, 2005). Herbalists who prepare and sell medicinal mushrooms or mushroom preparations often sell *G. tsugae* as Reishi or Red Reishi, and I have seen *G. lucidum* sold under the name Red Reishi as well as Reishi.

At times, this leads to confusion over which species is being purchased and questions about their medicinal properties. For the purposes of this book, I have combined *Ganoderma lucidum* and *G. tsugae* in discussions of description, medicinal components, and use. I separate the species in terms of habitat and ecology but treat them as indistinguishable with regard to medicinal use. My rationale for lumping the two together is supported by recent studies on the genus (Wang and Hseu, 1995, and Moncalvo, 2005). According to Moncalvo, the section of genus *Ganoderma* that contains both these species is now recognized as a complex of closely related and difficult-to-distinguish species. Genetic analyses of *G. tsugae* from North America indicate that they are "very close to the true *G. lucidum* of Europe" (Moncalvo, 2005). Many examples previously cited as *G. lucidum* worldwide have been misidentified and represent one of several of these related species. According to Moncalvo, "This leads to the question of what is the Oriental Reishi? A non-exhaustive molecular survey of taxa labeled *G. lucidum* in Asia, including strains commercially cultivated for the production of tablets or teas, shows that this name has been largely misapplied and encompasses many distinct species."

Though I certainly cannot say that there is no difference in the medicinal components of these closely related species, it seems clear from the literature that they share many components. In New England, Varnished Conks that grow on hardwood are called *G. lucidum,* and Varnished Conks that grow on softwood, usually hemlock, are called *G. tsugae.* At least in Maine, medicinal products labeled Reishi and made with wild-harvested native mushrooms are generally made with fruiting bodies found on hemlock, as these are by far the more common. Those growing on hardwood are occasionally collected in Maine but are much more common south of the state, including central and southern New England. For the purposes of this book, both related species are referred to as Reishi, as this is the most widely accepted common name among those who use it as a health-promoting dietary supplement in the United States.

Description

Reishi mushrooms fruit on wood (or, rarely, on the ground from buried wood). Two to twelve inches wide, they rise from an irregularly shaped knob of pale flesh but soon become more or less shelflike with a distinct stalk. The cap is often fan- to kidney-shaped but somewhat variable, and tough or corky in texture but not woody. The upper surface of the cap is colorful, with a distinctively shiny-varnished surface that with age becomes dull with dust and/or spores. The color of the cap is predominately a deep mahogany red with pale cream-to-ochre on the freshly growing margins. A fully mature cap is uniformly colored. On rare occasion, the cap color appears as shades of dark blue-green to almost black.

The upper surface is wrinkled, with some concentric zonation, especially in young specimens. The margin of the cap is often enrolled. The stalk is somewhat slender to thick and blunt, up to one-and-a-half inches thick and variable in length to seven inches (or occasionally shelflike without a discernible stalk). The surface and the color of the stalk is the same as the cap.

The pore surface is white to pale-yellow and bruises a brownish red. The individual pores are minute, four to seven per millimeter, and typically occur in one layer. The spore print is brown, and as the mushroom matures, huge numbers of the microscopic brown spores are typically deposited on the top of the cap and the surface of surrounding plants, coating the entire area surrounding the mushroom a rusty brown (see photo on page 67).

These are annual fruits, growing for only one season, with reported rare exceptions. The dead conks will persist into and over the winter and can often be seen alongside emerging new fruit.

Note: As is the case with many bracket fungi, Reishi fruiting bodies are indeterminate in their growth. This means that they have no set size and shape and will continue to get larger in response to available nutrient resources and growing conditions. (Mushrooms in general are mostly determinate in their growth, meaning that they emerge from their substrate as a knob or button that contains essentially all the cells that will be present in the mature mushroom.) In an indeterminate mushroom like Reishi, cells are added along the leading edge of the expanding cap. If the cap grows into contact with an object—say, a stick or branch—it will grow around the object, essentially engulfing it into the fruiting body. This makes for some interesting sights, as it often appears that the plant grew through the mushroom rather than the opposite. It also means that a growing indeterminate mushroom is able to heal damage caused by nibbling animals or knife-wielding humans, if the growing conditions remain ideal. I have returned to a tree where I had harvested Reishi the previous month and found new, fully formed fruiting bodies attached to the cut stem base of a fruiting body removed earlier.

Occurrence and Habitat

Reishi appears as a solitary fungus or in groups on the base or the lower twelve feet of dead or living trees or, more commonly, on stumps or downed logs. These two *Ganoderma* are considered butt-rotters, meaning their mycelium colonizes the major roots and the base of the trunk of the host and not the upper trunk or branches. This distinction fades when the mushroom is growing on logs on the forest floor. The mushroom will occasionally fruit from roots along the surface of the ground. Determination of the species is best made by the identity of the host as softwood/conifer (*G. tsugae*) or hardwood/broad-leafed (*G. lucidum* or *G. curtisii*). *G. lucidum* most often grows on maple, while *G. tsugae* grows almost only on hemlock. I have found *G. tsugae* fruiting on spruce, but by all accounts this is quite rare. An initial flush of fruiting bodies may start growth in the first warm weeks of late spring or early summer in New England and will continue to grow in size through-out the summer. Additional fruit may start growth at almost any point throughout the summer in response to wet periods, but I have not seen prolific later flushes. From midsummer into autumn the mushrooms mature and release spores actively over an extended period of time.

Ecological Information

Reishi is a weak parasite and an aggressive saprobe on the host tree, producing a white rot that can render the wood quite soft over a period of time. *G. tsugae* fruits primarily on dead trees, with the first signs of mushrooms typically seen two or three years after the tree dies or, on a stump, after the tree is cut. On standing dead trees, it is not clear if the tree death is connected to the Reishi growth. I have occasionally seen Reishi fruiting from the edge of pileated woodpecker feeding holes on a live hemlock, and it is not unusual to see a large dead hemlock broken off eight feet to twenty feet above the ground and fruiting Reishi on the lower portion. Reishi will fruit on a large stump or tree trunk for several years before exhausting the food source. Occasionally I see fruit emerging from well-rotted moss-covered logs on the forest floor.

Edibility

Reishi is not generally considered edible, though I do know several avid myco-phagists (mushroom-eaters) who collect and eat Reishi just as the new growth is emerging from the trunk of the tree and before any color develops on the pale knobs. They describe it as quite good in the very young stage. Mature mush-rooms become quite bitter due to the buildup of the medicinally desirable ter-penes. I have always avoided eating Reishi at the young stage, preferring to allow the mushrooms to mature, when I can use them medicinally. Certainly slugs find the young mushrooms quite tasty and will vigorously attack the small, pale emerging Reishi. Once the distinctive reddish color develops, the tough, corky texture and bitter taste would convince even a hardy diner to seek more flavorful fare.

Look-alikes

Due to its distinctive varnished appearance, it would be difficult to confuse this complex of species with other conks. *G. curtisii* grows on hardwoods in the southern United States and is considered by some to be a variant of *G. lucidum*. *G. oregonense,* found in the northwest United States and New Mexico, is much larger and thicker and grows on conifers.

Folk or Traditional Medicinal Uses

Perhaps no other mushroom carries the mystique of Reishi, as it is known in Japan, or Ling Zhi, as it is known in China. It has been an indispensable part of folk medicine in both countries for more than two thousand years—indeed, perhaps as long as seven thousand years in China, according to some sources. Its other common names speak to the fame of this mushroom: Mushroom of Immortality, Ten-Thousand-Year Mushroom, Herb of Spiritual Potency (Hobbs, 1995, and Halpern and Miller, 2002). Several of these names refer to Reishi's reputation for promoting longevity and vigor. Prior to the success in cultivating this mushroom over the past twenty years, it was an uncommon-to-rare mushroom, in high demand and therefore quite expensive. Its traditional uses are many, as it has a reputation as a panacea. On a short list are liver ailments, including chronic hepatitis; nephritis; hypertension; arthritis; insomnia; bronchitis and asthma; and gastrointestinal problems and cancers.

Current Medicinal Uses

Scientific studies have confirmed that many of the claims attributed to Reishi are indeed within reason. Various compounds extracted from *G. lucidum* have succeeded in reducing blood pressure, blood cholesterol, and blood sugar levels. Extracted polysaccharides and proteanated polysaccharides, as well as crude mushroom extracts, have shown strong immunomodulating activity. Reishi's polysaccharide glucans and related compounds, as well as some of its triterpenes, activate immune effector cells such as macrophages, T-cells, and natural killer cells that in turn produce a variety of cytokines such as TNFs and interferons. The anticancer, antitumor, and anti-inflammatory actions triggered by Reishi and demonstrated in numerous experimental trials with cell cultures and

Summary of Immunomodulatory Effects of Reishi
(From Gao, 2004)

- **Monocytes** (cell lines): Polysaccharide extracts influenced release of cytokines, including tumor necrosis factor-alpha, with a varying response using different polysaccharide components.

- **Macrophages** (including mouse peritoneal and human cell lines): Polysaccharide components increased the proliferation and activity of macrophages and the associated release of immunoactive mediator cytokines.

- **T-lymphocytes:** In a variety of studies using human cell lines, polysaccharide extracts of *Ganoderma*, both crude and refined, stimulated the action of T-cells as evidenced by release of interferons, TNF-alpha, and interleukins. The proliferation of T-cells was also seen.

- **Natural killer cells:** Extracts of *Ganoderma* were shown to stimulate NK activity in the spleens of mice in a dose-dependent manner. In tumor-bearing mice, *Ganoderma* polysaccharides enhanced the cytotoxicity of NK cells in spleen cells.

- **Dendritic cells:** In a study using mouse DCs derived from bone marrow, the exposure to polysaccharides of *Ganoderma* promoted maturation of the DCs and initiation of a broader immune response as measured by the increased release of cytokines.

animal subjects and, more recently, in human clinical trials are based on this enhancement of host immune response. There is evidence that Reishi triterpenes have a direct cytotoxic action on cancer cells. (See the sidebar list of pharmacological effects for Reishi.)

The market for nutraceutical compounds containing Reishi is immense and increasing rapidly. A worldwide estimate of the value of *Ganoderma* products, based on available information (2003), is $2.5 billion (Chang, 2005). China creates and markets the most products; other major producers include Japan, Taiwan, Korea, and Malaysia. Worldwide, cultivated Reishi has far surpassed wild-harvested supplies for medicinal use. This is due to high demand and the relative rarity of wild-harvested fruiting bodies. Before commercially cultivated Reishi became common in Japan, Reishi was a medicinal mushroom reserved for the powerful, wealthy, and influential.

Pharmacological Effects of Whole Reishi Extracts in Vivo and in Vitro
(See Hobbs, 1995, or Gao et al., 2004)

- Analgesic
- Anti-allergic activity
- Bronchitis-preventive effect, inducing regeneration of bronchial epithelium
- Anti-inflammatory
- Antibacterial against staphylococci, streptococci, and bacillus pneumonia (perhaps due to increased immune system activity)
- Antioxidant, by eliminating hydroxyl free radicals
- Antitumor activity
- Antiviral effect, by inducing interferon production
- Lower blood pressure
- Enhanced bone marrow nucleated cell proliferation
- Cardiotonic action, lowering serum cholesterol levels with no effect on triglycerides, enhancing myocardial metabolism of hypoxic animals, and improving coronary artery hemodynamics
- Central depressant and peripheral anticholinergic actions on the autonomic nervous system, reducing the effects of caffeine and relaxing muscles
- Enhanced NK cell activity in vitro in mice
- Expectorant and antitussive properties demonstrated in mice studies
- General immunopotentiation
- Anti-HIV activity in vitro and in vivo
- Improved adrenocortical function
- Increased production of interleukin-1 by murine peritoneal macrophages in vitro
- Increased production of interleukin-2 by murine splenocytes in vitro

Areas of Research

Active research into the medicinal uses of Reishi is ongoing in several countries around the world. Leading the efforts are China, Japan, Korea, and the United States. Because of the broad range of bioactive compounds found in Reishi, research is ongoing in a number of areas with the potential for development of pharmacological products, including:

- Antibiotic activity against specific various bacteria
- Antiviral activity HIV, influenza viruses, herpes simplex virus type one
- Antitumor anticancer activity in many forms of cancer via immune stimulation
- Anticancer action via directly cytostatic compounds
- Immunosuppressive and anti-allergic action via inhibition of histamine release
- Antihypertension
- Liver protection
- Hypoglycemic effects in diabetic patients
- Cholesterol-lowering properties through the actions of steroids and polysaccharide fiber
- Lipid lowering
- Antioxidant activity through the lowering of hydroxyl free radicals

Active Components
Polysaccharides (more than one hundred different types identified)
    Beta-D glucans including beta 1,6 and beta 1,3 branching patterns
    Gamma-D mannans
    Heteropolysaccharides
    Glycoproteins or proteoglycans
Terpenes (well in excess of 200 terpenes isolated)
    Ling Zhi-8 protein (anti-allergenic, immunomodulating)
    Ganodermic acids, triterpenes (anti-allergenic agents, reducing cholesterol and blood pressure)
    Steroids (ergosterols)

Collection, Preparation, and Use
For use as a medicinal mushroom, collect only fresh, growing conks. The ideal time for collection is when the mushroom is at its full growth and actively dropping spores but before it has begun to deteriorate. This is generally in mid- to late summer, though is quite dependent on weather patterns. A good indicator is when the cap margin has turned the deep red of maturity from the lighter yellow of active growth. Old, dead, or dying fruits are prone to attack by molds, and an examination of the pore surface will usually show this. Discard any fruiting bodies showing evidence of mold, which renders them unfit for use and possibly toxic.

Unless I am using Reishi fresh in a tea or broth, I generally dry the mush-rooms as soon as I bring them in from the forest. They are fairly tough and much more easily sliced fresh than when dry, so I slice them into quarter-inch strips and dry them in a commercial dehydrator or on screens in a warm attic room. Follow-ing drying, put the Reishi into jars or heavy-grade freezer bags and place them into a freezer for at least twenty-four hours. This will kill off any small eggs of the prehistoric-appearing horned fungus beetle (*Bolitotherus cornutus*), a common pest on *Ganoderma*. If left in place, the larvae of the beetle will hatch in the spring or summer and merrily consume your dried Reishi supply.

Preparations of Reishi, both commercial and those made at home, are gener-ally based on hot-water extracts or double-extraction tinctures made with a com-bination of ethanol and hot-water extractions (page 125). The polysaccharides and proteins are water-soluble, but not all of the terpenes and steroids are effectively extracted with water. In addition, the fruiting bodies can be dried, ground into a powder, and taken in capsule form or mixed into teas or juice. In general, I would suggest an initial cooking to assist in the breakdown of cell structure to release the active components. The fruits are tough, making grinding quite a task.

To prepare a simple tea at home, place a half cup of dried mushrooms, cut or broken into pieces as small as possible, into two quarts of cold water and gently bring the mixture to a simmer or low boil. Simmer for at least 20 to 30 minutes and then strain the tea, squeezing out the liquid from the remaining solids. Drink a small cup of the resulting tea, hot or cold, at least daily. It will be quite bitter, and you might want to add it to juice or dilute with additional water. Refrigerate extra tea for future use.

Reishi is often found as one component of a mixture of mushrooms and/or herbs in a preparation. I make a mixed double-extraction tincture of Reishi, Turkey Tail, Birch Polypore, Maitake, and Chaga for broad immunostimulating impact. Many Traditional Chinese Medicine preparations include Reishi, especially those used to stimulate immune function or to provide liver protection.

Chapter 8

Maitake *(Grifola frondosa)*

Common names: Hen of the Woods, Maitake, Sheep's Head (PHOTOGRAPHS ON PAGES 68–69)

R elatively few health-promoting mushrooms get as much attention from researchers, the media, and history as Maitake. It is in the top tier of medicinal mushrooms, due to the progress made in researching its anticancer abilities and the fact that human clinical trials indicate that the species promotes immunomodulation. I first knew *Grifola frondosa* as Hen of the Woods, and for years my goal in collecting this bountiful mushroom was purely gastronomic.

Shortly after moving to Maine in 1981, I got to know my friend Mark Digirolamo and to appreciate his gentle nature and encyclopedic knowledge of birds, plants, and much else in the natural history field, including mushrooms. In the fall of 1982, when I was exulting over the discovery of my first Hen of the Woods, Mark told me about a Digirolamo family tradition. When he was a child, his Italian grandmother would buy "nasce" in a South Philadelphia market to make a type of marinated mushroom pickle with garlic, Italian spices, and good olive oil. According to Mark, *nasce* referred both to the mushroom, *G. frondosa,* and to the dish she made of it. Mark was interested at my news and told me about a developing crop of *Grifola* he and his then-girlfriend Beth were watching so they could pick the mushrooms when they were just a bit larger. As almost all wildcrafters know, you never reveal the location of your natural treasure trove, but over time, and in response to increasingly detailed questions, it became clear that I had discovered and harvested "their" Hen of the Woods. Thus began a long friendship and competition revolving around Maine's abundant mushrooms.

Maitake is a great edible mushroom. In a survey I conducted in winter 2007–08 of seven hundred mushroomers in New England, *G. frondosa* was the third most popular of the wild mushrooms. Only Chanterelles and Black Trumpets exceeded its popularity as an edible. Easy to recognize and wonderful to eat, it is relatively common in areas of New England with plentiful oaks.

Description

Maitake fruits as a large cluster of overlapping caps arising from a many-branched, fleshy central stalk. A mature cluster can range from six inches to well in excess of two feet in diameter. Average weight is four to seven pounds, and commonly exceeding twenty pounds. Weights in excess of a hundred pounds have been reported, though the largest I have seen in New England was approximately forty-five pounds. Each individual cap is one-half to three inches wide, spoon-, fan-, or tongue-shaped, usually with a wavy margin. The flesh of the cap is about a quarter-inch thick, with a firm yet pliable texture. The overall cap color can vary from pale gray to almost charcoal, or light tan to chocolate brown and somewhat mottled. Occasionally I have found clusters that are almost white, especially those growing in the absence of light. The compound stalk terminates as a lateral attachment to each cap. The upper cap surface is generally minutely roughened to somewhat fibrous. The pore surface is white, aging to somewhat yellowish; individual pores are one to three per millimeter and somewhat angular. The spore print is white.

Occurrence and Habitat

Hen of the Woods can be found on the ground near its host tree or, rarely, growing on the wood of a well-decomposed hardwood stump. I find it most often associated with an over-mature oak (red oak in our area), but occasionally it grows on beech, ash, or, reportedly, other hardwoods, and even on softwood trees. In Maine, Hens fruit any time after the first of September and can be found until early November in a mild autumn. Fruiting is triggered by the first few late-summer nights when temperatures fall into the fifties, and while rainfall is a factor, fungi like Maitake, with the huge biomass of mycelium growing in a large tree trunk, are less affected by dry periods. On living trees, it normally produces fruit every other year. On dead trees, however, it commonly produces several to numerous fruiting clusters yearly for several years. I suspect that, on a dead tree, the fungus does not expend energy overcoming host defenses and can grow more rapidly through the host wood and therefore fruit more heavily. I have seen as many as twenty-three individual clusters fruiting simultaneously around the base of a single massive live red oak. In general, the more individual clusters there are, the smaller each will be.

Hen of the Woods is common throughout those areas in the Northeast where large oaks occur in any number. Common in the Midwest as well, it is rare in the Southeast and the Northwest, and essentially absent on the West Coast and in the arid Southwest (Arora, 1986). In rural New England a hundred years ago, much of the countryside consisted of small farms with a patchwork of fields and pastures surrounded by stone walls. Today, thousands of miles of these stone walls can be found deep in forests that have grown back as nature has reclaimed abandoned farms. In many of these forests, the largest trees are found along the old walls, massive specimens of oak, maple, hemlock, and others. These matriarch oaks are the perfect age for Hens, and I follow the walls scouting for them. When I find a productive tree, I make note of the exact location for future years. As my friend and fellow mushroom-seeker Kerry Hardy says, "Think of running a trapline of Hen trees as you check known sites and areas of good potential. Not all the traps will be productive in any one year, but over time all will continue to produce."

It might be only one tree in a hundred that has a Hen, but once found, it is like money in the bank. If you find a Hen tree fruiting, note the exact location for future foraging; you will kick yourself if you lose it. Mr. Hardy very believably claims to be intimately acquainted with seventy-five or eighty Hen trees.

Ecological Information

Hen of the Woods is a saprobe, or weak parasite, attacking the heartwood of the tree and causing it to rot over time. Along with other mushrooms that grow on the larger roots and lower trunk of the tree, it is known as a butt-rot fungus. Its primary food source is the lignin and cellulose of the heartwood. It can live on a tree for many years without causing major discernible damage, though clearly throughout this time it is slowly rotting the tree, weakening the roots and lower trunk and increasing the risk of wind-fall. I return now to the story of finding my first Hen in 1982. I have been collecting fruit off that same red oak for more than twenty-five years, and though the tree is now quite hollow, the branches are fully leafed out.

Maitake reluctantly gave up the secrets of its cultivation, and since the mid-1980s has been available in cultivated form in markets around the world, initially in Japan and China and more recently in the United States. Maitake is cultivated outdoors on logs or, more commonly, indoors on sawdust in climate-controlled mushroom fruiting rooms. Success in cultivating "exotic" mushrooms such as Maitake and Lion's Mane has made these tasty and health-promoting species easily available year-round in many areas of the country.

Edibility

Maitake rests solidly on the list of my favorite five edible mushrooms. I have great respect for the medicinal value of Maitake, but my true regard is led by my stomach and gastronomic discernment. Pound for pound, few mushrooms can compete with Maitake for taste, texture, and versatility in cooking options. My wife, Valli, loves this mushroom as much as I do; her favorite healthy mushroom dish is Maitake sautéed with garlic and tamari over a bed of organic basmati rice.

Nutritionally, Maitake is around 27 percent protein by dry weight and is a source for Vitamins B1 B2, C, and D, and niacin. The fruiting body contains iron, magnesium, calcium, and, especially, phosphorus. Analysis of beta glucans content showed a level of 14.5 percent of dry weight (Stamets, 2000).

Caveats: Maitake, like almost all wild mushrooms, *must* be cooked prior to eating. It is difficult to digest raw, as a former neighbor discovered. Having heard many stories of gastronomic pleasures told by satisfied Maitake consumers, she was quite excited when I offered her a cluster of Maitake one fall day. She took it home and planned on cooking it for dinner, but during the day, as she moved through her house, she began breaking off pieces and eating them raw. Several hours later she became quite sick to her stomach, as her system rejected what it could not break down. The sickness lasted only as long as it took to clear her system.

On the long road to approval as a licensed drug in the United States, Maitake D-fraction, one of Maitake's most promising extracts, was tested for any negative effects. In a monthlong controlled trial with healthy subjects, no negative side effects were noted (Glauco et al., 2004). In 1998, the FDA approved an Investigational New Drug application from Maitake Products, Inc., of New Jersey, to conduct phase 2 clinical trials using Maitake D-fraction on advanced breast and prostate cancer patients. In consideration of previous Maitake research, the FDA authorized skipping a usual first-phase toxicity study and going directly to the second phase.

Look-alikes

There are several other clustered ground-dwelling polypores. *Grifola (Polyporus) umbellatus,* another edible medicinal, is smaller, with all of its rounded caps coming off a central stalk. Berkely's Polypore (*Bondwarzwei berkelyii*) is another clustered ground-fruiting mushroom that reaches impressive sizes at the base of large oaks. It normally fruits earlier in the season, is cream-tan in color, and does not develop the spoon-shaped caps. Though considered edible when young, it has reportedly caused gastrointestinal distress in some people. *Meripilus sumstinei (giganteus),* known as the Blackening Polypore, while rare in Maine, is more common farther south and occupies the same habitat as Maitake, fruiting at the base of oak trees. Its notable feature is the tendency to bruise black where the pore surface is touched and to blacken with age. This mushroom is also edible when young, though I have never tried it.

Folk or Traditional Medicinal Uses

The longest history of Maitake use is in Japan, where it has been popular as a medicinal mushroom for hundreds of years. Prior to the 1980s it was available in Japan and China to only a few industrious collectors and those wealthy enough to afford it. In many parts of the world, Maitake is uncommon in nature and all the more valued due to the scarcity.

Current Medicinal Uses

Maitake for medicinal and culinary use is easily available as fresh fruiting bodies in season or cultivated year-round. It can also be purchased for medicinal use as dried, powdered fruiting bodies or mycelium in capsule, tablet, or bulk form. The mushroom can be easily tinctured as a way to release the medicinal components. There has been an increase in Maitake fractions sold as trademarked proprietary compounds that contain one or more of the mushroom's many potentially useful active components. It is these licensed proprietary compounds that are being used in the clinical trials for Maitake and that make up the majority of the research carried out in cell culture and animal studies.

Antitumor: Maitake fractions are currently being tested in phase two human clinical trials in the United States for treating several forms of cancer, including breast and prostate. These tests are needed for FDA approval and to determine the optimal dosing for use of mushroom extracts. The ongoing study will examine the immune-activating effect of Maitake on tumor size, clinical symptoms, and quality of life.

In several human clinical trials conducted using whole mushrooms and/or fractions extracted from the fungus, it has been shown that Maitake resulted in improvement of symptoms by 58 percent (liver), 68.8 percent (breast), and 62 percent (liver) in patients with second- to fourth-stage cancer. In those patients with leukemia, brain, or stomach cancer, symptoms improved by less than 20 percent (Lindequist, 2005).

In numerous studies using animal subjects or cell tissue cultures, a proprietary glucan fraction and whole fruiting bodies have demonstrated antitumor/anticancer properties through the indirect action of stimulation of macrophages and T-cells and the resultant increase in TNFs, interferons, and interleukins. Mice with tumors that were treated with Maitake D-fraction showed marked increase in the production and activity of NK cells with direct cytotoxic effect on tumors (Kodama et al., 2005).

Maitake D-fraction was tested with cell cultures of human bladder cancer and showed strong growth reduction after seventy-two hours. When it was combined with Vitamin C, the effect was a 90 percent cell death rate (Konno, 2007), suggesting a synergistic interaction between Maitake extracts and Vitamin C.

Cancer preventive: In one study designed to test the potential for Maitake as a cancer-preventing agent, mice injected with a cancer-causing substance were then fed on a diet including differing concentrations of Maitake D-fraction. The control group did not receive Maitake. It was shown that the Maitake group developed cancer at a significantly lower rate than the control group.

Immunostimulating: Early on, Maitake was shown to stimulate a host's immune system through the action of polysaccharides present in both the mycelium and the fruiting body of the fungus. The increased immune response has supported the assertion that medicinal mushrooms such as Maitake can help prevent or reduce opportunistic infections and cancerous growths. Studies with laboratory mice show that the immune stimulation is due to the activation of macrophages, T-cells, and NK cells (Namba et al., 1992).

The D-fraction of Maitake was shown to increase activity of NK cells by triggering increased production of a chemical messenger called interleukin-12 (IL-12) by immune system macrophages (Kodama et. al., 2005). In turn, IL-12 activates the NK cells.

Mice fed with polysaccharides extracted from Shiitake (50 percent), Maitake (25 percent), and Reishi (25 percent) demonstrated increased thymus and NK cell activity as well as increased activity of macrophages. (Yin et al., 2007). This study suggests that the addition of mixed mushrooms to the diet could increase the immune function, at least in mice. A similar trial with mice using mycelium and culture broth of Maitake as a portion of their diet showed increased activity of phagocytic cells without adverse signs of inflammatory response (Wang et al., 2008).

Chemotherapy side-effect reduction: In a trial with mice, the use of Maitake increased the response by immunocompetent cells to boost the immune system following treatment with chemotherapy agents for cancer (Kodama et al., 2005). This suggests that in stimulating immune response following the immune-suppressing side effects of chemotherapy, Maitake may mediate the negative side effects of such therapy in cancer patients.

Maitake MD-fraction has been shown to have a dose-dependent effect on the bone marrow cells of mice, with an increase in the production of colony cells and granulocytic macrophage colonies (Lin et al., 2004) in these cells following the administration of Maitake MD-fraction. The increase in these types of cells and cell chemicals are signs of an immune system recovering from the effects of an immune depressant such as chemotherapy.

Antiviral: Maitake contains a number of glucan polysaccharides that have been shown to stimulate the human immune system. In addition, these compounds have been shown to have an inhibiting action on several viruses, including HIV (Lindequist et al., 2005).

In cell cultures, Maitake D-fraction in combination with human interferon markedly increased viral replication inhibition in the hepatitis B virus (Gu, Li, Chao, 2007).

Blood pressure regulation: Studies of spontaneously hypertensive rats have shown that dried fruiting bodies added to the diet of the test animals resulted in lowered blood pressure. An uncontrolled, non-randomized trial with hypertensive human adults showed a decrease of 7 percent in systolic, and 9.4 percent in diastolic, blood pressure following the ingestion of 1,500 milligrams of mushroom extract twice daily (Hobbs, 1995).

Cholesterol lowering: In studies with rats, a high-fat diet containing dried Maitake showed a significant lowering of the amount of high-density lipids (HDL) and cholesterol in the bloodstream of animals compared to those fed a normal diet, due to a greater degree of cholesterol excretion in feces (Fukushima et al., 2001).

Hypoglycemic antidiabetic effects: Early research using Maitake for tumor control and prevention showed that for some people Maitake had the unexpected side effect of lowering their blood sugar. This is being looked at as a positive effect with diabetics and others with hyperglycemia. Studies with mice and rats show a clear positive impact on lowering blood sugar levels. In a study using rats, orally administered Maitake mycelium significantly decreased serum triglyceride and blood glucose levels as compared with a control group (Lo, Hsu, Chen, 2008).

An alpha-glucan fraction of Maitake significantly decreased the body weight, level of fasting plasma glucose, glycosylated serum protein (GSP), serum insulin, triglycerides, cholesterol, free fatty acid, and malondialdehyde (MDA) content in livers (Hong, 2007), possibly because Maitake increases the sensitivity of insulin receptors.

An initial case trial in humans with type 2 diabetes showed that regular use of a polysaccharide fraction of Maitake could enable the patients to control blood sugars without other medication (S. Konno et al, 2001, and Lindequest, 2005).

Areas of Research

Ongoing phase 2 clinical trials with Maitake are exploring its effectiveness with prostate and other cancers. Clinical trials utilizing Maitake to address blood sugar regulation are ongoing.

Active Components

Polysaccharides
    1,6 branched beta-D glucans
    1,4 branched beta-D glucans
    1,3 branched beta-D glucans
    Hetero-beta glucans
    Acidic beta glucans
Ergosterol derivatives (Vitamin D2)

Collection and Preservation

Hen of the Woods often fruits in one big flush. But this is not a mushroom that comes up overnight and is gone by sundown the next day. In the cool fall weather, I have watched as a just-emerging young cluster slowly matures into its prime over the course of ten days, and when I picked it, there were still days to go before it became less than excellent. In warmer, dry weather, the clusters grow and mature more quickly, though there are still many days to maturity. A cluster growing in full sun can quickly dry out in the absence of rain. A tree, especially a dead tree, that fruits early in the fall can produce a second crop later on. When the flush comes, there can be several to many clusters, all calling out to be turned into great meals and health-promoting preparations. It is very easy to become greedy when you are faced with as much as fifty pounds of mushrooms from one large tree.

Try to collect the mushrooms when they are almost fully mature, i.e., with the spoon-shaped caps fully expanded but before the pore openings become obvious, and certainly before the pore surface yellows with age. A younger cluster is fine, but if you can wait, do so. This also allows you to pick a couple of young clusters for your use and return later for more.

Unlike many other edible mushrooms, Hen of the Woods is not usually infested by the larvae of fungus flies except during particularly warm fall weather; if this occurs, carefully cut away the parts with the telltale tunnels before cooking.

Maitake is a choice edible and well suited to being cut into small, bite-sized pieces, then sautéed or parboiled and frozen.

Preparation and Use

Maitake should be a part of a regular diet as a great-tasting and healthy funtional food. It is available year-round in many co-ops, health food stores, and supermarkets. Some of these sources even employ organic methods of cultivation. Wild Maitake can be found in the fall and either dried or frozen for future use. The harvest from one tree can easily supply a family for the winter. I prefer to either sauté or blanch chopped Maitake and then freeze it in serving-size portions. Most years my freezer is stocked with twenty or more quart freezer bags packed with enough for one meal for the family. Just like my friend Mark, Northern Italians commonly pickle this mushroom in olive oil, vinegar, and savory spices after parboiling. Cooking starts to break down the cell wall components, making the bioactive polysaccharides more available.

Dried fruiting bodies can be easily ground to a powder in a blender or food processor and kept in a sealed glass container. Some care must be taken with a dried, fleshy fungus to protect it from insect damage. Powdered Maitake can be added easily to soups, broth, gravy, or other cooked foods. Capsules of dried or powdered Maitake can be taken twice daily as an immunostimulating dietary supplement. I have used a preparation of dried Maitake as the main ingredient of an immune supportive broth for people undergoing chemotherapy.

Sold as dried fruiting bodies, capsules of fruiting body and/or mycelium powder, or extracts in a liquid or powdered form, Maitake is becoming increasingly available as a dietary supplement. Several proprietary extracts are marketed, including Maitake D-fraction and Maitake MD-fraction.

Chapter 9

Turkey Tail *(Trametes versicolor, Coriolus versicolor)*

Common names: Turkey Tail, Kawaratake (Japan, "Riverbank Mushroom"), Yun Zhi (China, "Cloud Fungus") (PHOTOGRAPHS ON PAGES 70–71)

Each year I teach a dozen or more mushroom identification classes and lead numerous walks and talks devoted to wild and medicinal mushrooms. On almost every occasion there are people for whom mushrooming is an entirely new pursuit, even a new concept. Often one of these newcomers will contact me in the next few days or weeks, exclaiming at the numbers of mushrooms they are seeing on their walks in the woods and the diversity of forms, colors, and habitats they are discovering. Often they suggest that it must be an incredibly productive year.

In reality, they have had their eyes opened to the fact that mushrooms are living in their world, and like magic, they suddenly see them in numbers they never imagined. Such is the power of our mind that until we are made aware of the existence of something, we are unable to see it.

This holds especially true for Turkey Tails. Ubiquitous, common, and prolific, Turkey Tails are also unassuming, diminutive, and understated. Once people learn to notice Turkey Tails, I can assure you they will see them in almost any forest in this country, to say nothing of forests the world over. Though their colors and pattern of growth can be striking and incredibly variable, Turkey Tails are also somewhat muted, and their pattern can blend into the forest's background clutter. Yet this forest-dweller is arguably the best known and most researched (by western medical standards) of all the medicinal mushrooms. It is also among the easiest to find and use.

Description

The Turkey Tail assumes the classic bracket fungi appearance. It forms multiple overlapping shelves of leathery mushrooms that can cover a host trunk or log and persist throughout the year (see photos on page 70). A thin-fleshed, leather-textured fruiting body is always found growing on wood. Each fruiting body is kidney- to fan-shaped, ranging from three-quarters of an inch to four inches wide, but commonly fused together to form overlapping rows or shelves with a smooth to wavy margin. Growing on a horizontal surface or the top of a downed log, the Turkey Tail can develop a rosette-shaped body with the appearance of overlapping

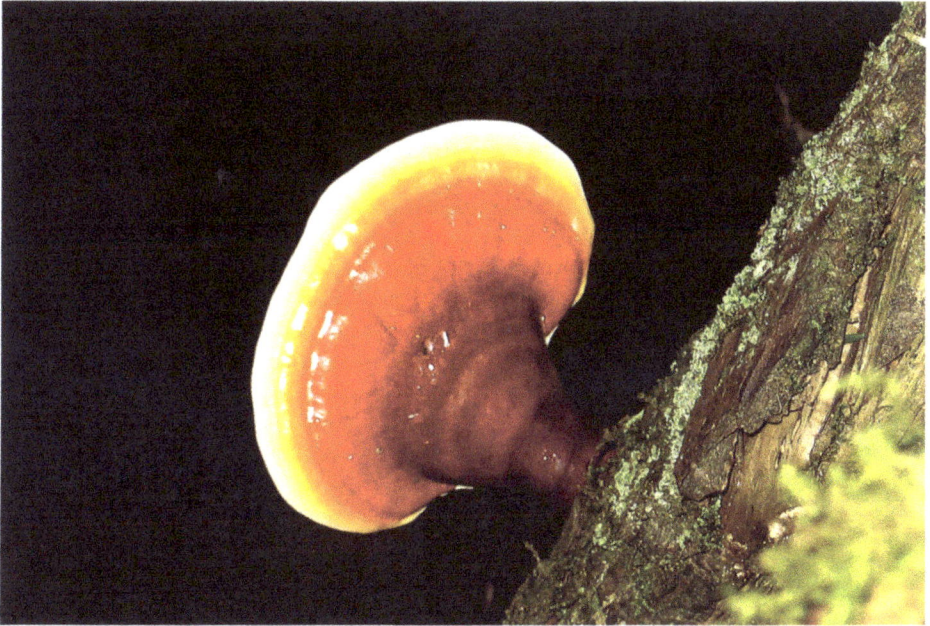

A young Reishi

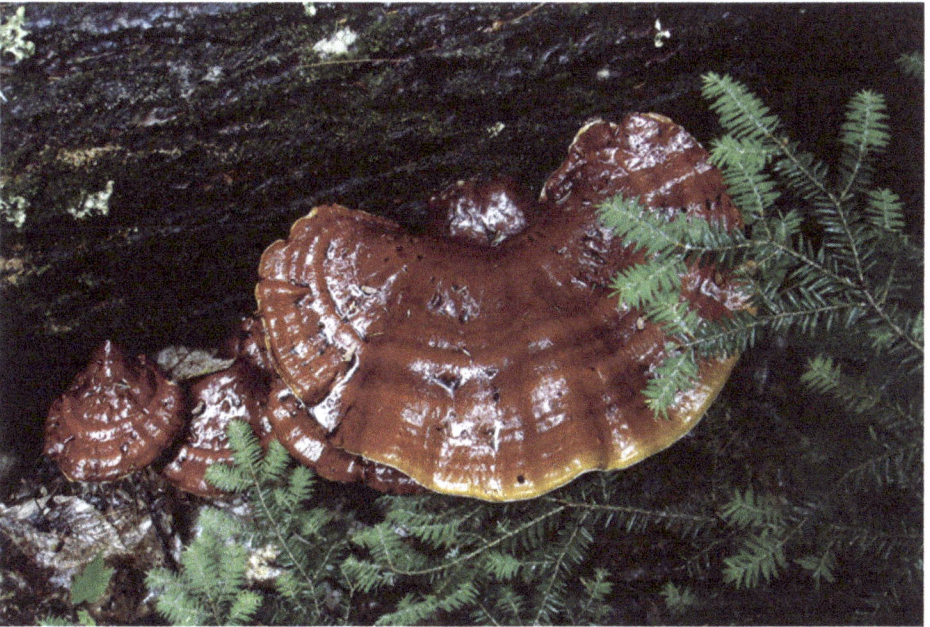

Mature Reishi fruiting bodies can vary considerably in size.

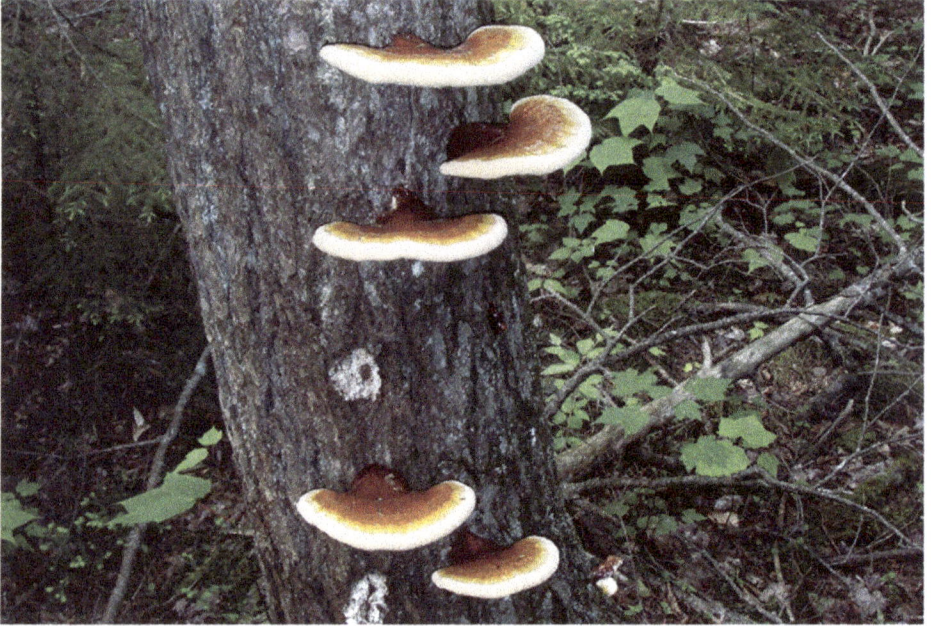

Reishi on a hemlock trunk

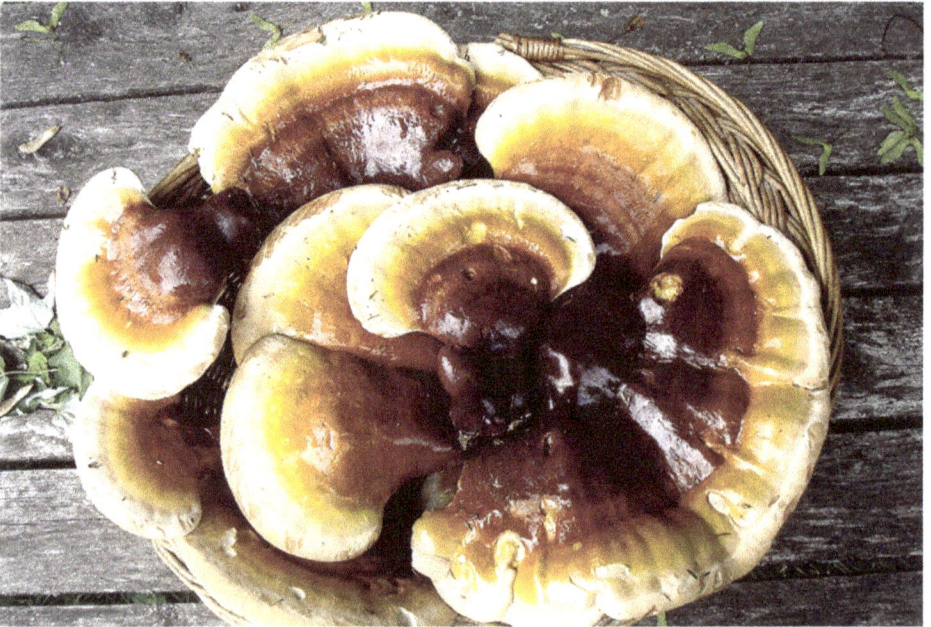

A harvest basket of Reishi

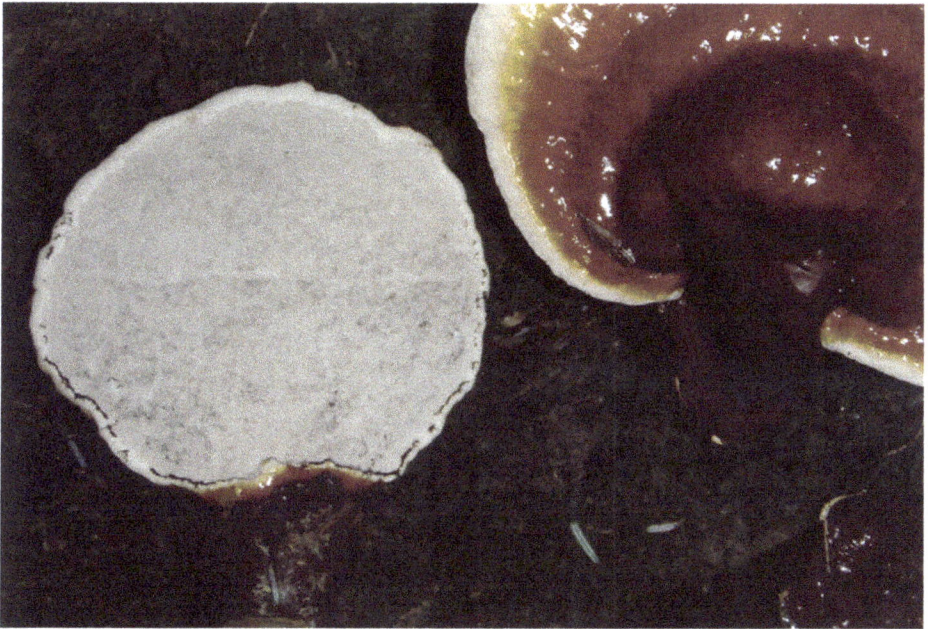

On left, the underside of a Reishi

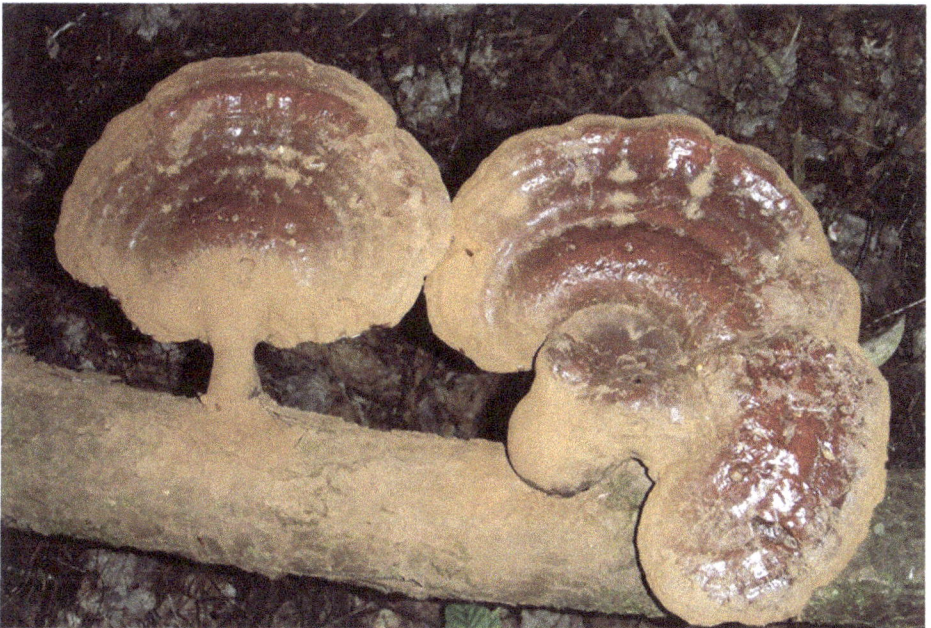

Reishi fruiting bodies release spectacular amounts of brown spores.

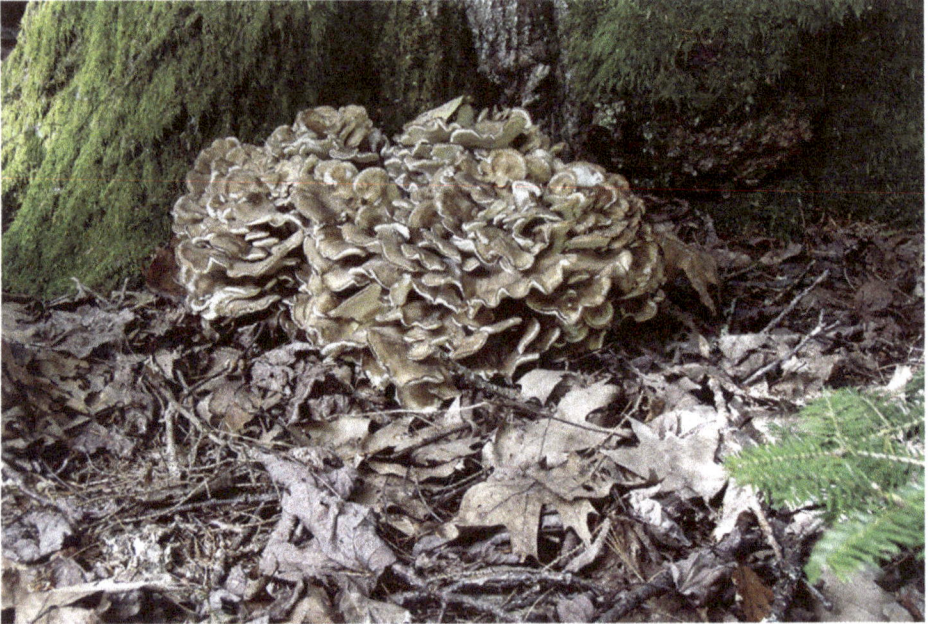

Maitake, or Hen of the Woods, on the forest floor

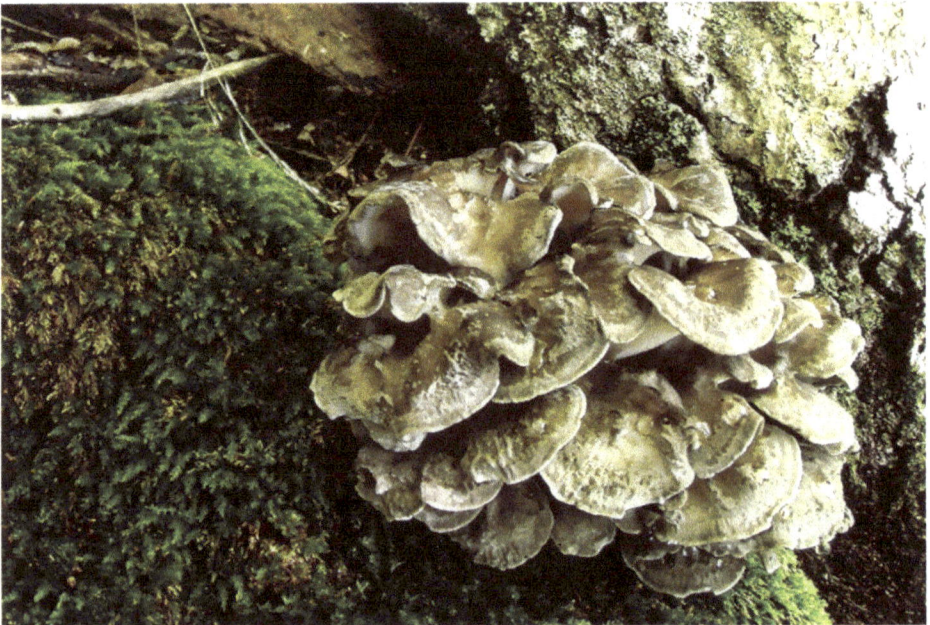

Maitake fruiting from beech wood

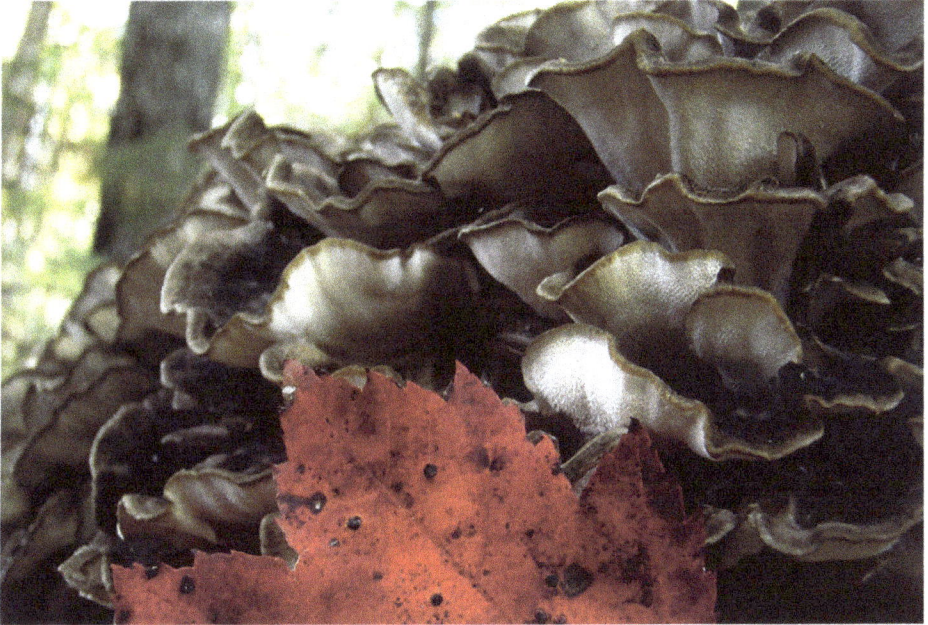

Pore surface of Maitake

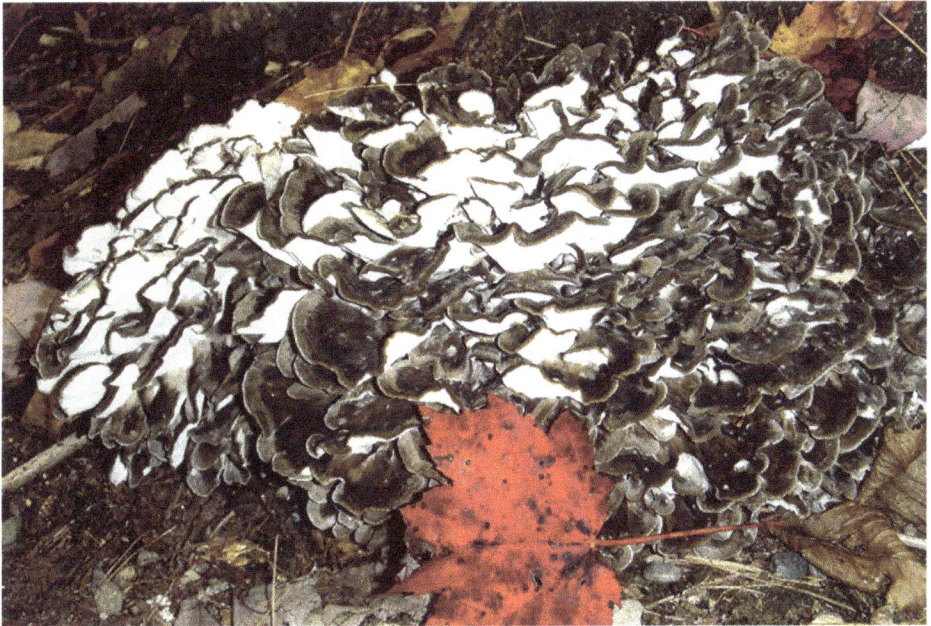

Twenty-five pounds of Maitake!

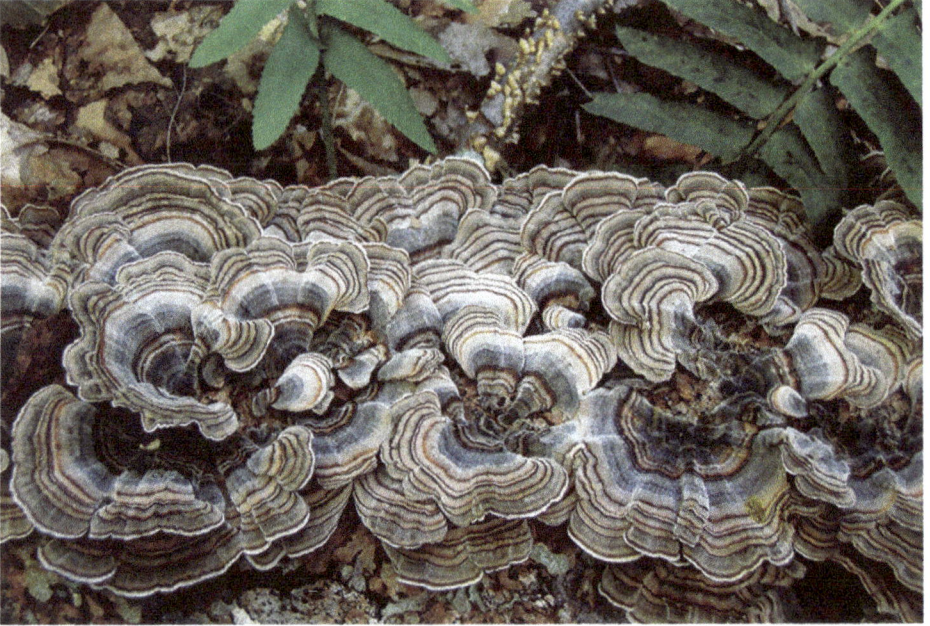

Above and below: The color of Turkey Tails can vary from brown/tan to gray/blue.

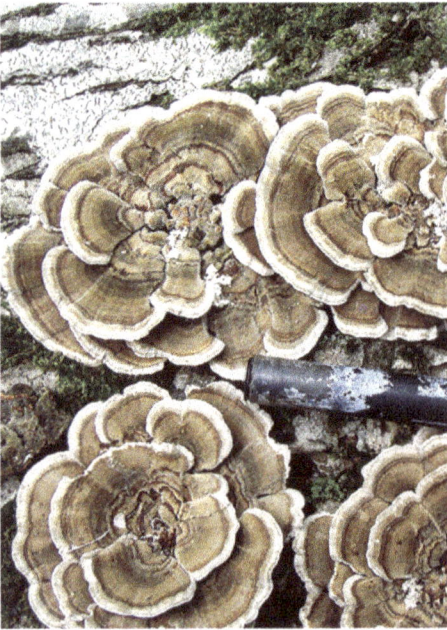

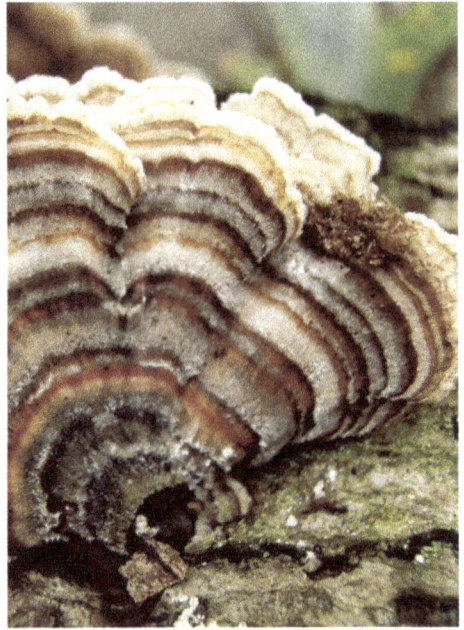

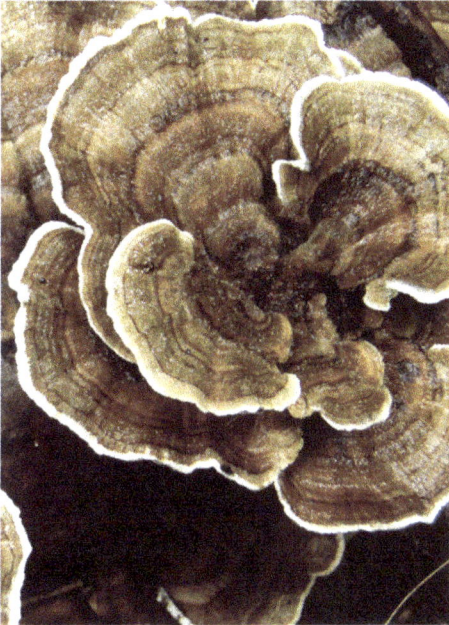
White outer edges show active growth.

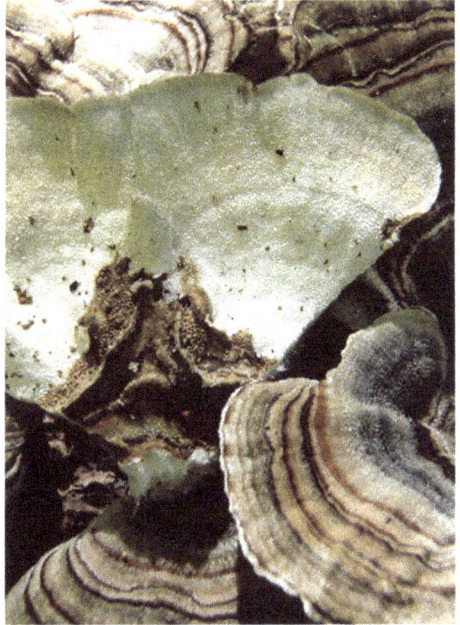
Turkey Tail, underside

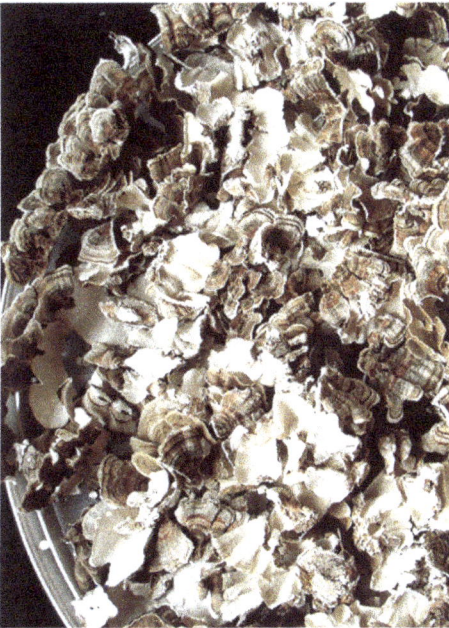
Turkey Tails ready to be simmered and processed

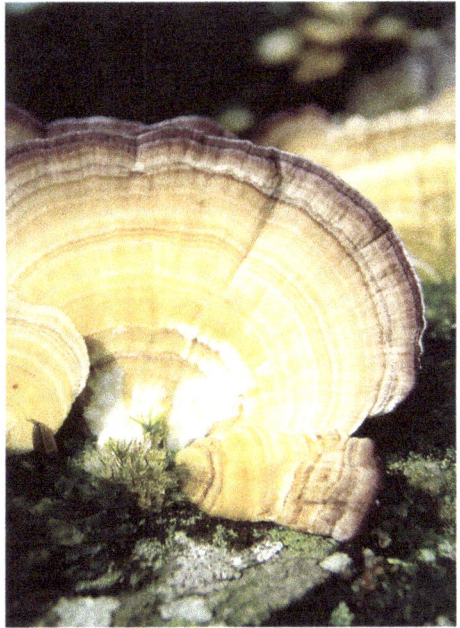
The Violet-toothed Polypore resembles Turkey Tail.

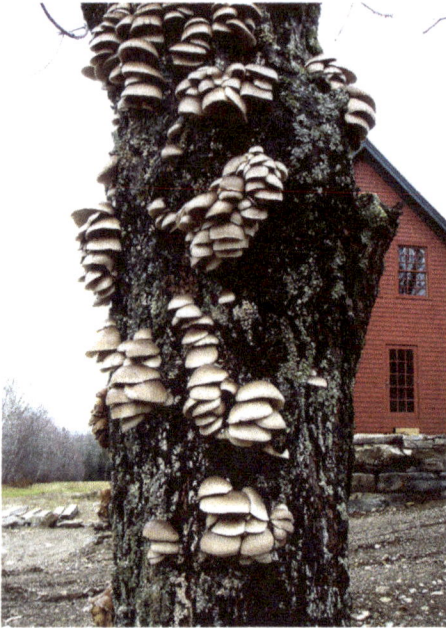

Prime Oyster Mushrooms on sugar maple trunk

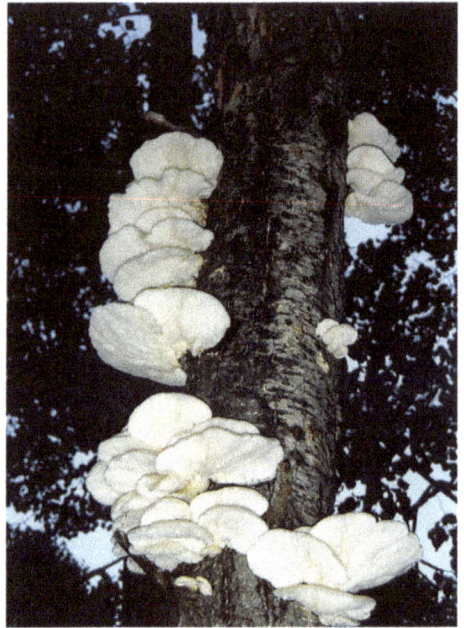

Oyster Mushrooms on poplar, showing the white gills

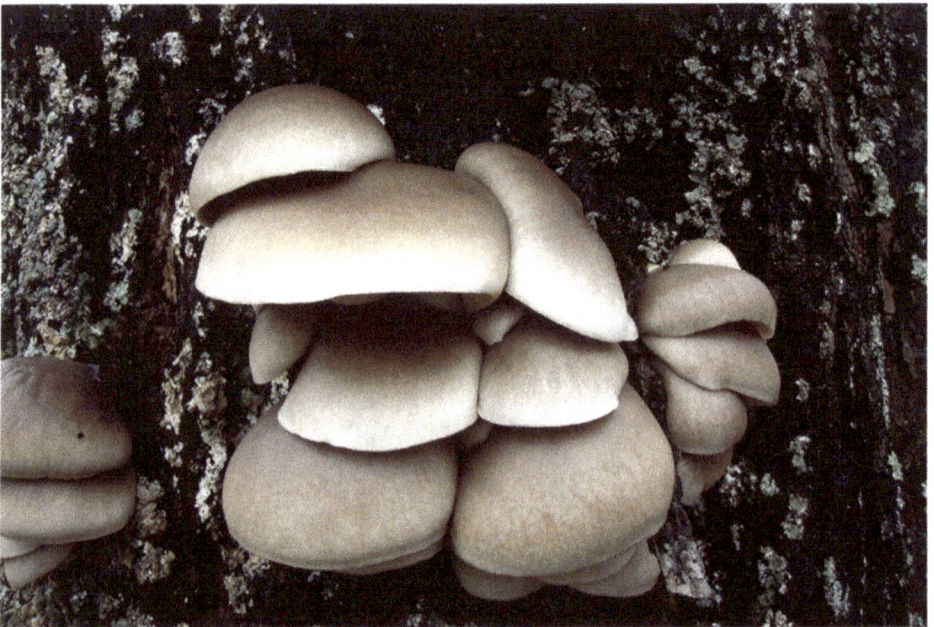

Oyster Mushrooms in mid-autumn

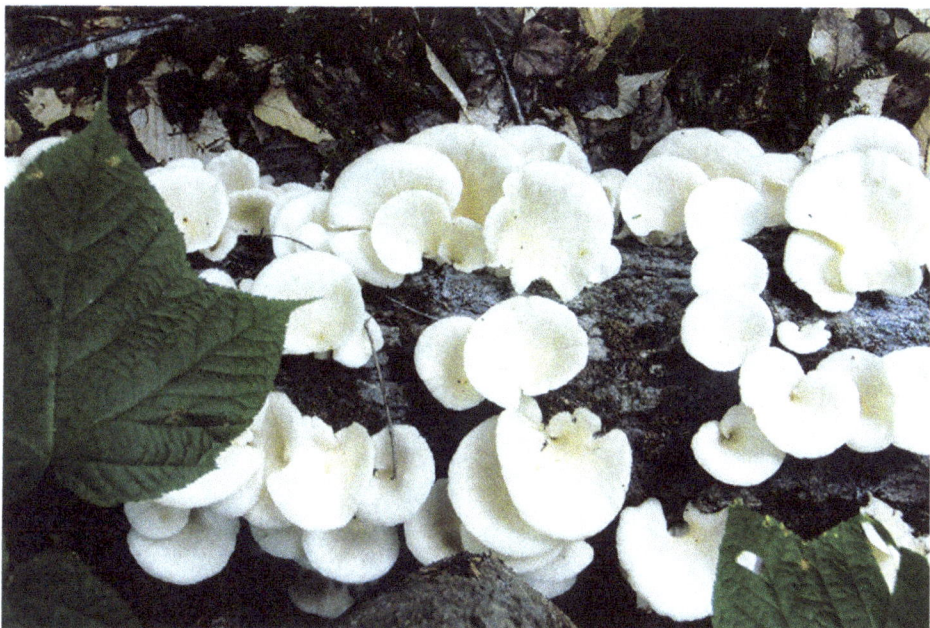

When growing on a horizontal surface, such as a downed log, Oyster Mushrooms often assume a funnel shape.

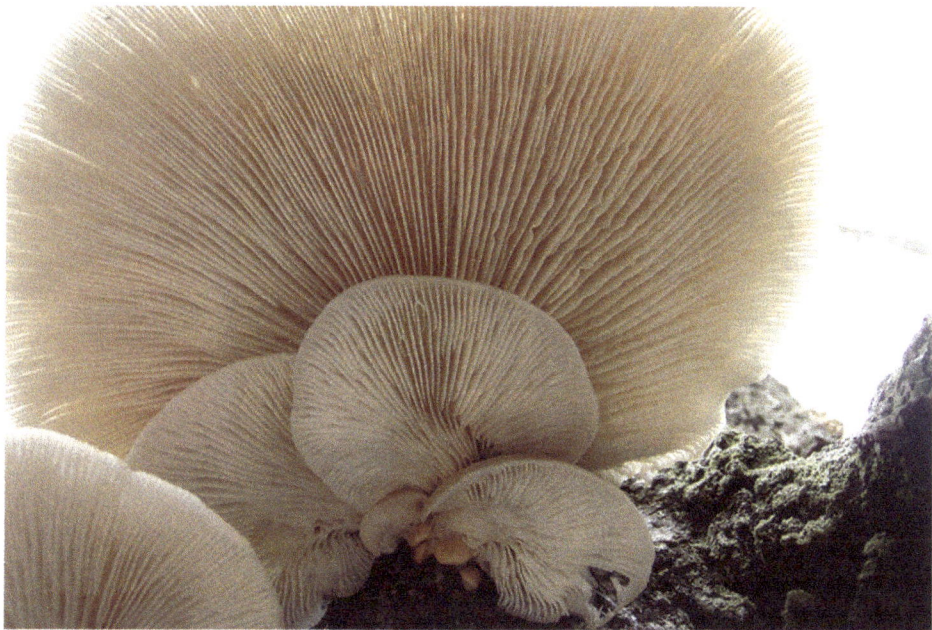

Close-up view of gills on Oyster Mushrooms

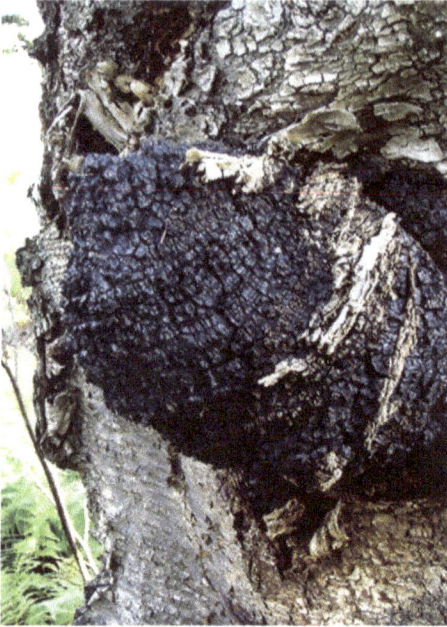

Bits of bark and outer layers of wood can be caught up in an expanding Chaga sclerotium.

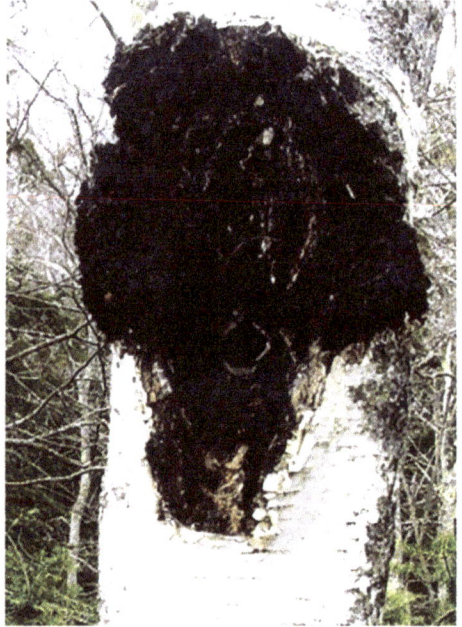

Chaga with woodpecker hole

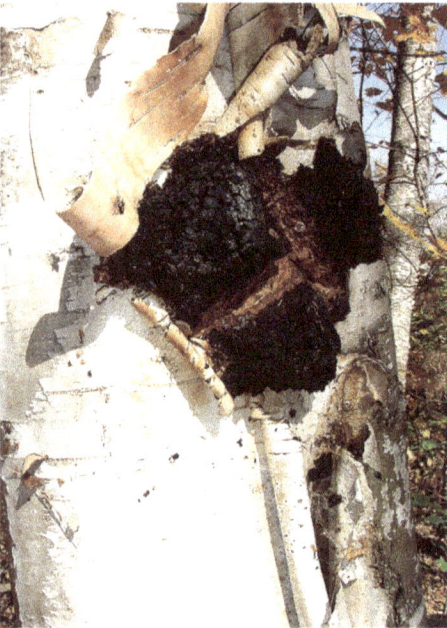

Chaga on white birch

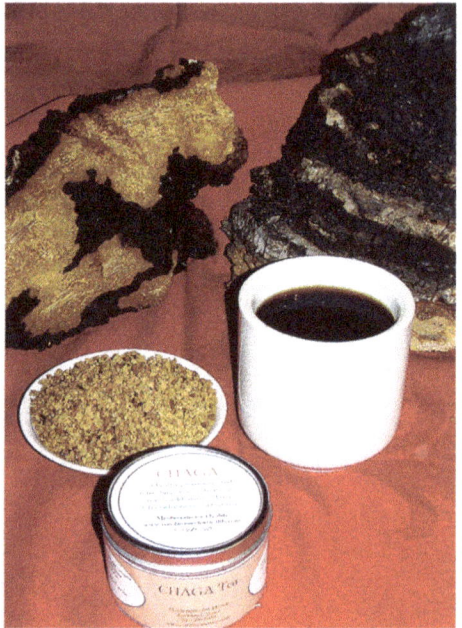

Foreground: Ground dried Chaga and Chaga tea. Background: Chaga sclerotium, underside (left) and upper side (right).

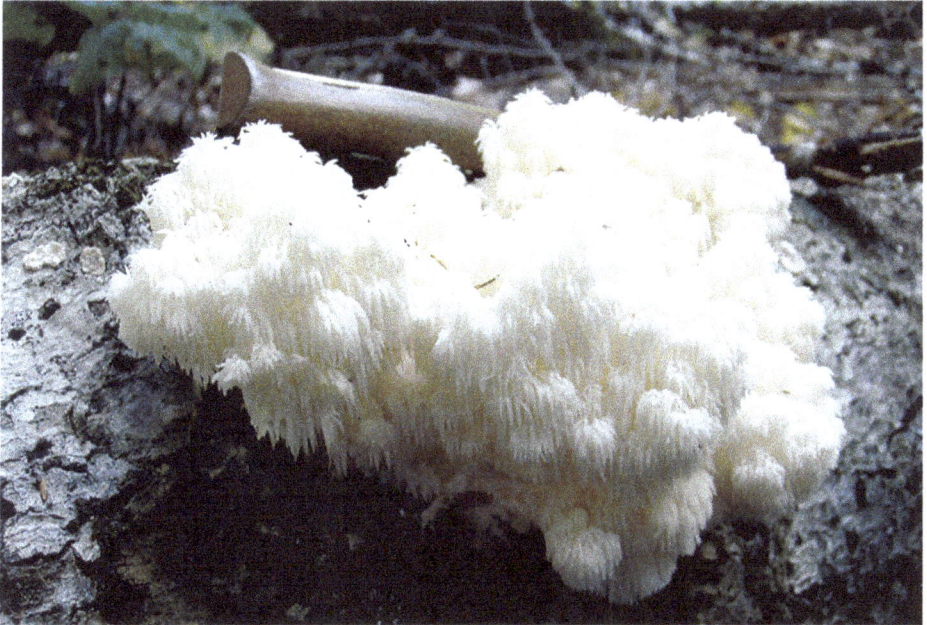

Pure white Lion's Mane gleams in the shadows.

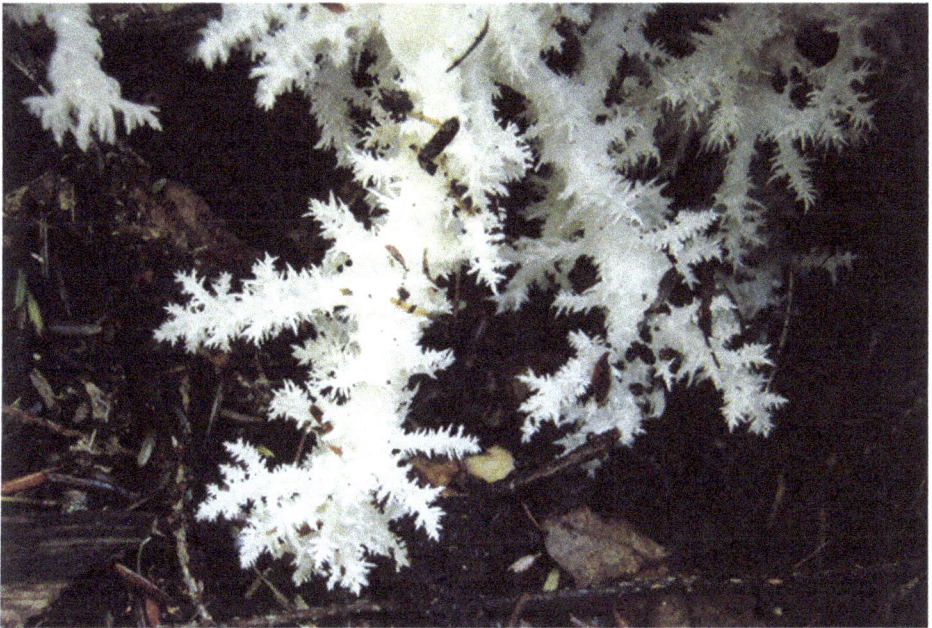

Lion's Mane showing the branching pattern observed on some specimens

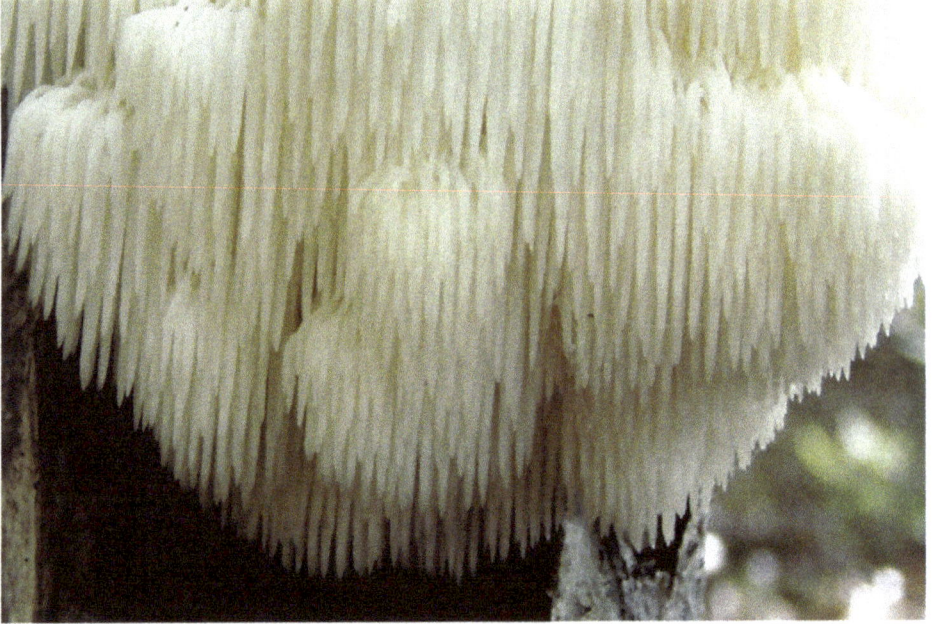

Hericium americanum is often more dense than the closely related *H. coralloides.*

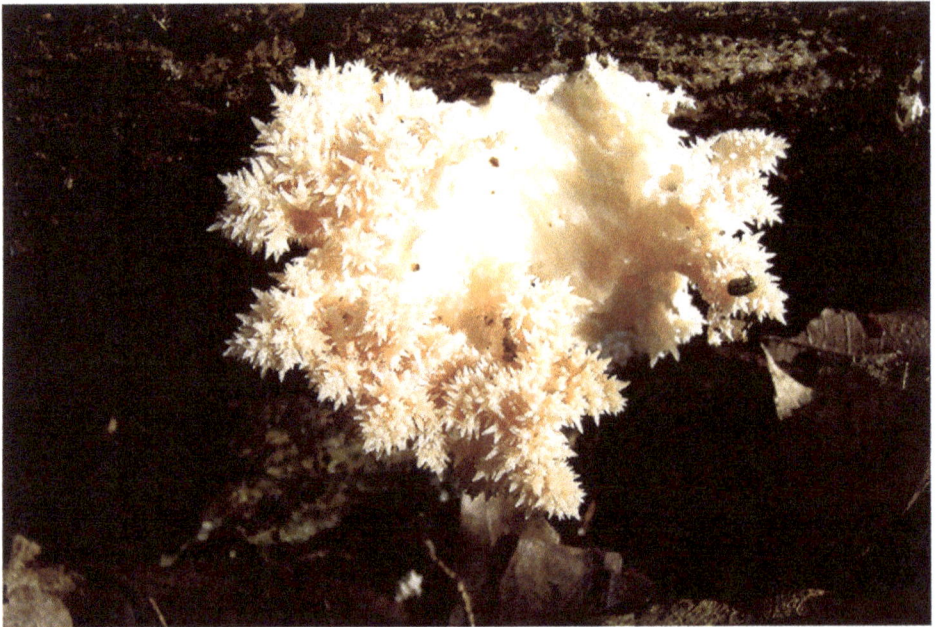

A young specimen of Lion's Mane showing pink hues

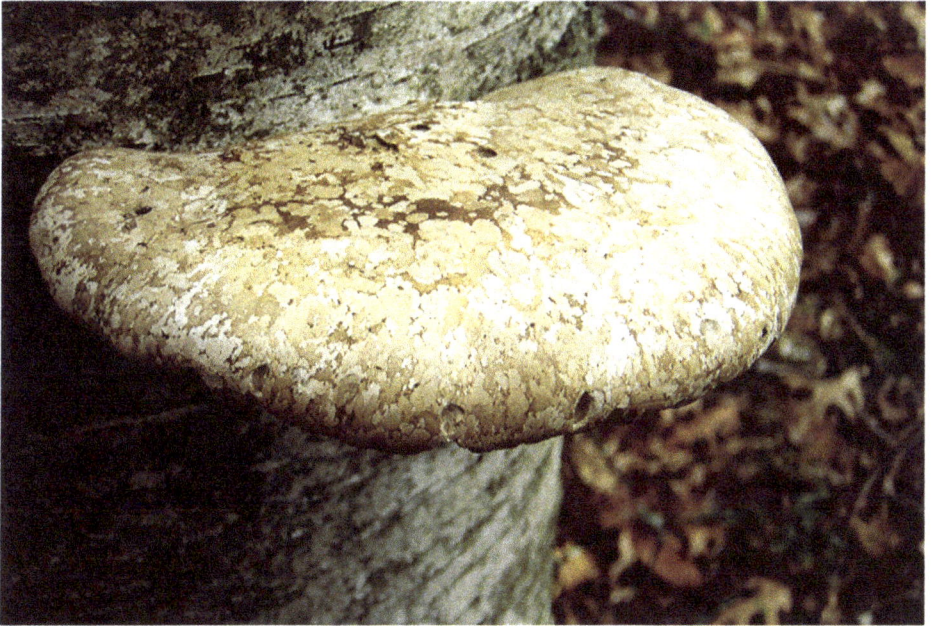

A mature Birch Polypore

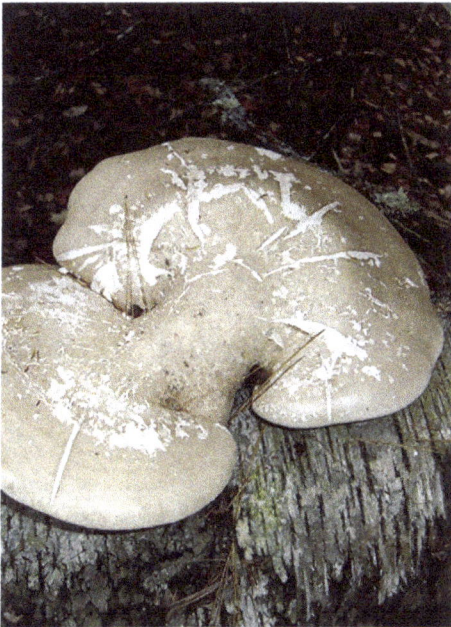

Birch Polypore on a downed log

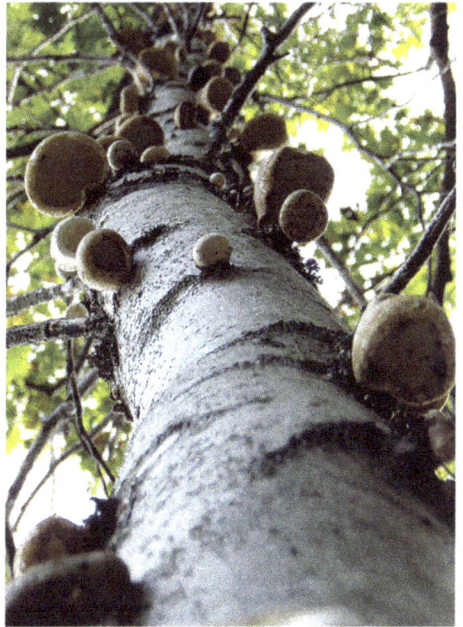

Fruiting bodies marching up the trunk of a dead tree

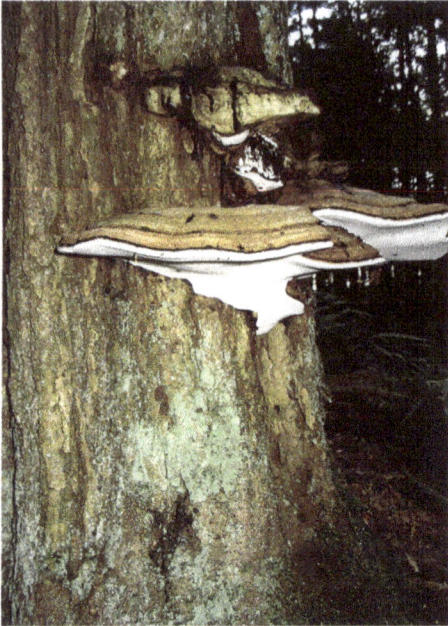

A large Artist's Conk

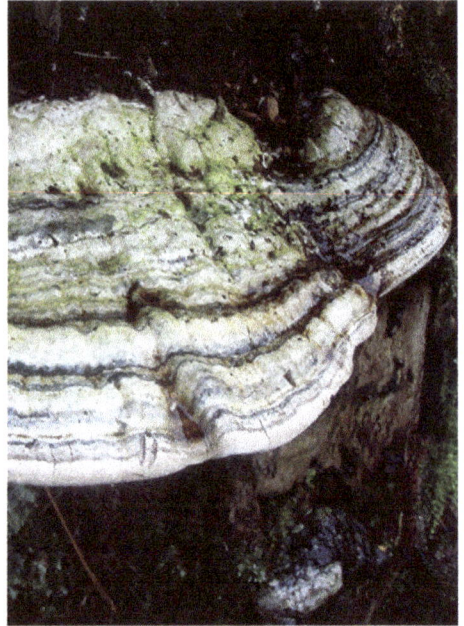

Concentric growth rings on upper surface of Artist's Conk

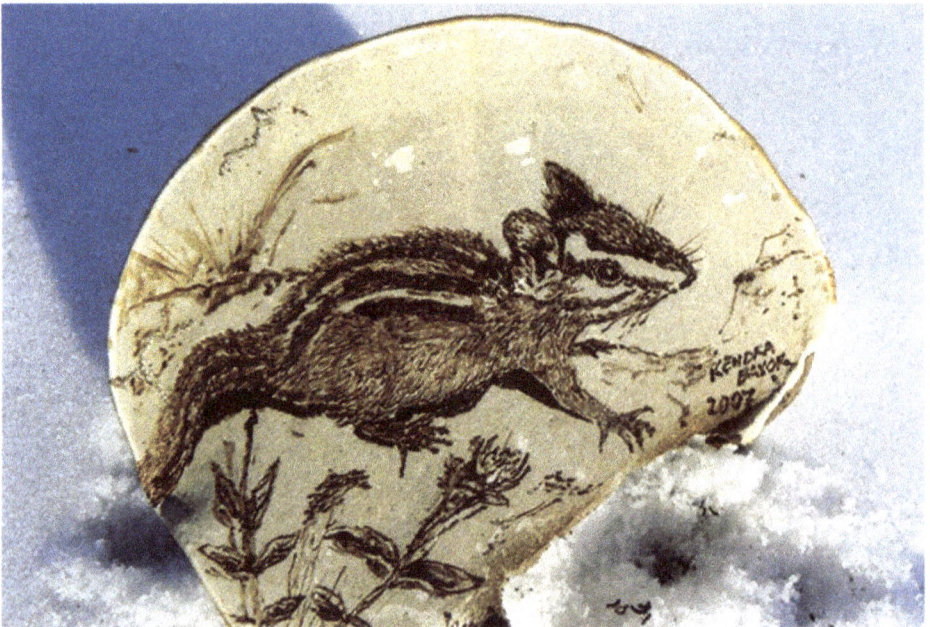

The firm, white undersurface makes a fine etching canvas for artists. Photo by Kendra Bavor.

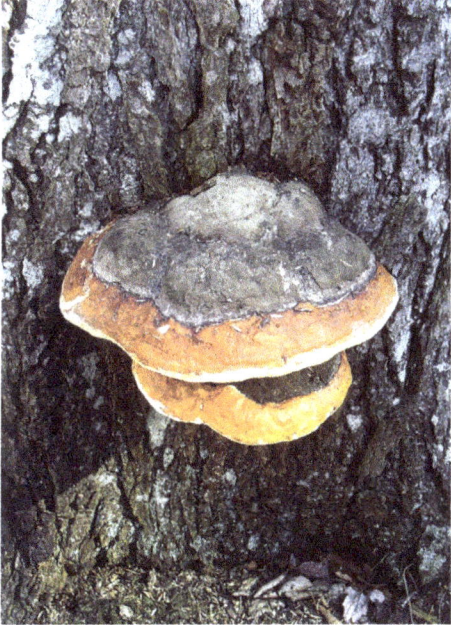

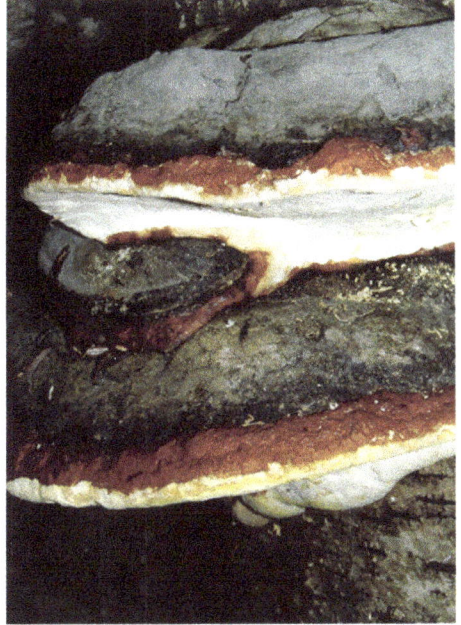

Above and below: The color and width of the red "belt" on Red-belted Polypore varies.

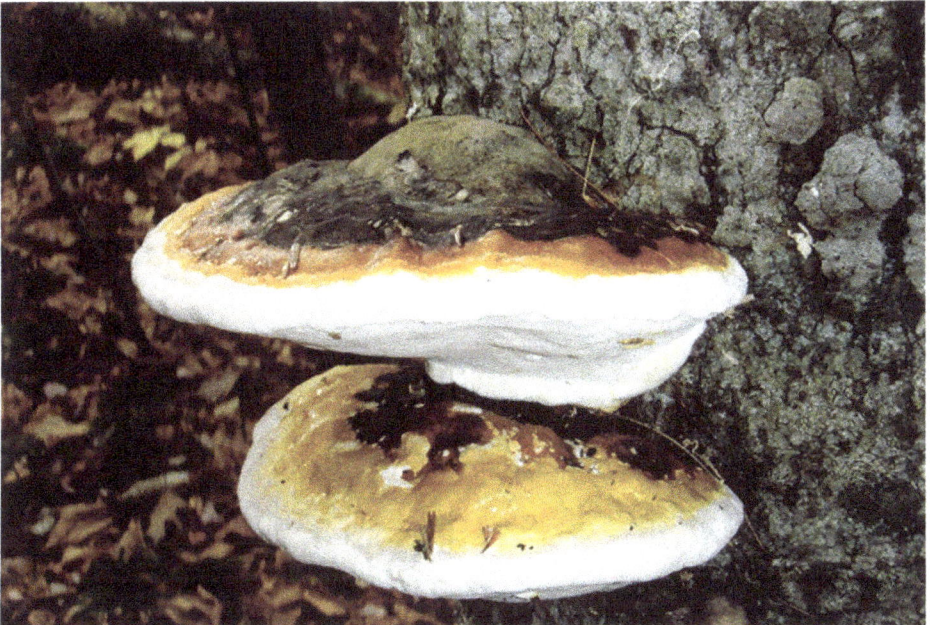

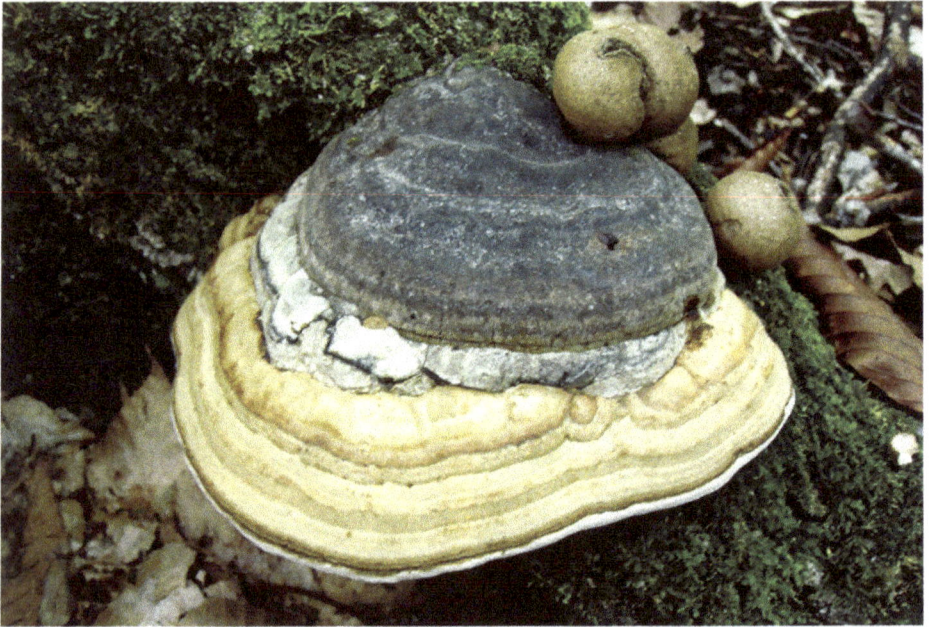

Older gray and younger tan growth rings show clearly on this Tinder Conk.

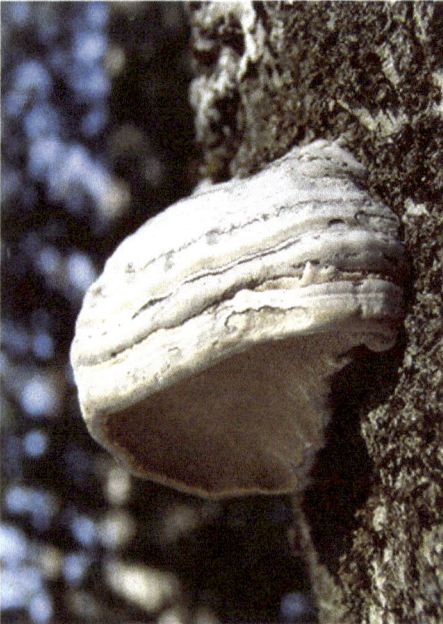

Pore openings on a small Tinder Conk

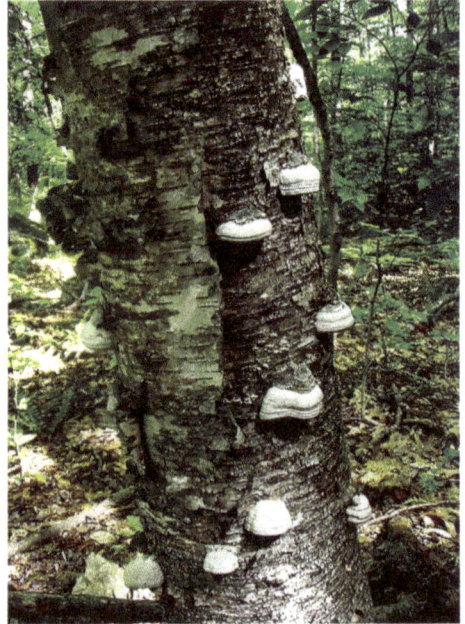

Tinder Conk grows mostly on dead wood, such as this birch.

"petals." The upper surface of the caps is alternately silky and hairy with each color shift. The individual caps are only three millimeters thick. The upper surface is distinguished by concentric bands of alternating contrasting colors, varying from white to tan to reddish-brown, gray, and almost black. Occasionally shades of gray will alternate with dark gray-blues; hence the name Turkey Tail. The underside of the cap is white to pale yellow and consists of minuscule pores (three to five pores per millimeter) with rounded to angular openings. The spore print is white to slightly yellow, though it is frequently quite a challenge to get enough spores deposited to see the spore color.

Occurrence and Habitat

Turkey Tail is one of the more common small, leathery polypores. It grows prolifically in clusters, rosettes, rows, and overlapping tiers on the trunks, cut stumps, and downed wood of a wide range of hardwood trees and shrubs, the most common being oak, beech, maple, and birch. It has also been known to colonize conifers, in rare instances. The persistent fruiting bodies can be seen throughout the year, but the active growth and fruiting body formation is in the late summer and fall, after which the fruiting body dies back and is replaced by a new one the following year. Turkey Tail grows in more tropical climates as well, where the growth cycle is not as curtailed by the changing seasons. If you seek this species in New England, look for it in a hardwood forest that has seen logging activity over the previous few years. The fungus actively colonizes the stumps of cut hardwoods and will fruit with vigor for several years. You would be hard-pressed to find a stand of hardwoods not graced by this beauty.

Ecological Information

The Turkey Tail is a prolific white-rot saprobe that breaks down the lignin and cellulose in dead wood. It is not unusual to see many contiguous feet of overlapping leathery shelves of Turkey Tails where the fungus has completely colonized a log or a dead standing tree trunk. It can also be found as a weak parasite on living trees where a wound or other injury has opened the bark to attack. The complex of species that make up *Trametes,* along with a few other small bracket fungi, are among our most common and visible forest fungi.

Edibility

The Turkey Tail is nonedible and nonpoisonous. The leathery texture precludes any gastronomic possibilities. The fruiting bodies are used in a hot-water decoction for health reasons only with the fungus removed prior to drinking the broth.

Look-alikes

A number of small, leathery shelf fungi grow on the sides of logs or on standing timber. These include other species of *Trametes*, including *T. conchifer,* which is similar but smaller and with pale colors, and *T. hirsute,* which as the name implies is hairier and also pale in color. *Trichaptum biformis,* the Violet-toothed Polypore, is similar in form but with a paler cap and pores that become tooth-like and have a violet tinge (photo on page 71). It is the other very common leathery and small-bracket fungus that colonizes hardwood logs along with the closely related *T. abietinus,* which grows on conifers. None of the similar-appearing species has been reported as toxic, and none of the look-alikes has any known medicinal value.

Medicinal Uses

Turkey Tail is the best-researched and most clinically tested of the medicinal mushrooms, at least by allopathic medicine standards. In the mid-1960s, a Japanese chemical engineer saw his neighbor succeed in using the mushroom known there as Kawaratake as a traditional remedy for his cancer. The engineer's initial horror at the idea that his friend would rely on an unproven treatment to address his cancer turned into wonder and intense interest in the mushroom behind this folk remedy. He then worked on a team that tested Kawaratake for antitumor activity, isolated a highly active strain of the fungus, and extracted and concentrated a bioactive fraction from the fruiting body. The licensed fraction is a group of protein-bound polysaccharides called Polysaccharide-Kureha, now known as PSK or by the trade name Krestin. The Japanese Ministry of Medicine initially approved it for use in treating cancer in 1977 (Hobbs, 2004). Since that time, *T. versicolor* has been the subject of many studies, initially with cell line cultures and animals and then in substantially more than three hundred clinical trials with human patients. Unlike many earlier studies of other medicinal mushrooms, some of the clinical trials using *Trametes* have been double-blind, using controls without treatment and a study group taking the mushroom extract. Individual subjects in a double-blind study do not know if they are in the control or the study group.

Beginning in the 1980s, Chinese scientists began a program of testing numerous strains of *T. versicolor* for bioactivity. Eventually they chose one very active strain, Cov-1, and began testing a polysaccharide-protein fraction of the strain, which they licensed under the name Polysaccharide P (PSP). Numerous studies of the Japanese PSK and the closely related Chinese PSP have been published. Experimental studies using human cell cultures, animal trials, and, later, human clinical trials have been carried out, using Turkey Tail components or simple hot-water decoctions. The two main proprietary fractions have been marketed for sale as commercial anticancer drugs in Japan, China, and other Asian countries. They are available in the United States as a dietary supplement.

PSK is the second leading anticancer "drug" in Japan and is responsible for several hundred million dollars in sales annually throughout Asia, where both PSK and PSP are recommended for use as adjunctive therapy, along with chemotherapy or radiation therapy. Under these conditions they have been shown to strongly inhibit cancers, improve survival times, and help conserve or improve the immune status of patients facing the toxic stresses of conventional treatments (Kidd, 2000). PSK and PSP have also been shown to be effective adjuvant treatment along with chemotherapy or radiation for a number of cancers, including gastric, esophageal, colorectal, breast, and lung (Fisher and Lang, 2002). Both fractions are effective when taken orally and are also administered by injection.

At this time in the United States, phase 2 clinical trials using PSK as a treatment component in several forms of cancer are under way as PSK moves through the rigorous process of FDA approval as a licensed medicine.

Folk or Traditional Medicinal Uses

Turkey Tail has been used as a folk remedy in Japan and China for hundreds, if not thousands, of years. Traditionally, fruiting bodies of *T. versicolor* have been harvested, dried, ground, and simmered in water as a tea. This type of extract is recorded in the Chinese edition of *De Materia Medica* as treatment for a variety of symptoms associated with liver dysfunction and respiratory-tract infection, and for promoting a healthy body and spirit generally (*Compendium of Materia Medica*, vol. 28). Over the past century, the extract has been best known in Japan for use as an adjunct in the treatment of gastric and colorectal cancer. It was this type of use that prompted Japanese scientists to investigate the healing properties of Turkey Tail, leading to the isolation and production of PSK.

Current Medicinal Uses

Immunomodulator: Extracts of Turkey Tail are best known as compounds that stimulate the action of a number of immune system components to increase immune response. Turkey Tail fractions consisting of glucans and glucan-protein complexes, crude and licensed, used in vitro or in vivo, stimulate increased response in a range of immune and inflammatory cells. The immune cells known to possess receptors for and to be activated by Turkey Tail proteoglucans include bone marrow cells, NK cells, neutrophils, monocytes and macrophages, DCs, and T- and B-cells. These cells are activated through the release and action of a number of chemical messengers and mediators, including cytokines and chemokines. Once activated, they increase the body's ability to identify and remove or destroy either invasive cells or the body's own cells that have become malignant. This same effect has been shown as an effective method to address the needs of patients with depressed immune functioning (Zhang et al., 2000). Some of the specific ways these cells respond include:

Dendritic cells are located throughout the body, concentrated in places such as the skin, mouth, and gut where they are most likely to come in contact with invasive organisms. They are designed for the early detection of invasive or malignant cells when they begin to mature and set in motion the body's response to invasion. PSK from Turkey Tail has been shown to concentrate in DCs shortly after ingestion (Kidd, 2000), supporting the idea that the mushroom polysaccharides are treated as potentially invasive organisms by the body. Once the DCs are triggered, they moves to lymph nodes, where they stimulate the action of other immune cells such as T-cells. PSK has been shown to reverse or counteract the suppression of DC activity in patients with cancer (Kanazawa et al., 2004).

Neutrophils and **macrophages** both act with direct cytotoxicity against foreign or malignant cells, including bacteria, viruses, and cancer cells. Several studies have shown that PSK from Turkey Tails stimulates the activity of neutrophils and macrophages toward enhanced cytotoxicity against cancerous cells and to inhibit metastasis in tumor-bearing mice and rats.

Cytokine modulation: Cytokines are chemical messengers that trigger a maturation or transformation of leukocytes and other immune cells. Some are also directly cytotoxic against cancerous cells. Examples include any number of interferons, interleukins, and TNFs. Aqueous extracts of Turkey Tail have been shown to stimulate or restore production of a number of cytokines that act in turn on other immune effector cells (Hobbs, 2004).

Antitumor and anticancer effects: In Japan, as mentioned before, PSK is an approved anticancer medicine available by physician prescription. In China and many other countries of the world, PSK and PSP are sold over the counter as an approved adjuvant treatment for a number of cancers and also used as a general immune builder and cancer preventive. *Trametes versicolor* has been tested in clinical phase 1, 2, and 3 trials, primarily in Japan and China, and has shown positive effects with a number of cancers, including increased survival rates, increased disease-free periods following surgery, and reduced metastasis. The types of cancers where Turkey Tail has proven significantly effective include colorectal, lung, breast, gastric, esophageal, nasopharyngeal, and leukemia.

Immunotherapy with Turkey Tail extracts has been shown to have the greatest impact when used in conjunction with chemotherapeutic agents. Under these circumstances, in addition to the increased survival rates and reduction in cancer resurgence and metastasis, the mushroom extracts also reduced the negative side effects of the chemotherapy agents. The immunostimulating effect also enables treatment in those individuals whose depressed immune functions would otherwise prevent effective treatment (Fisher and Yang, 2002).

Antimicrobial: Though extracts of Turkey Tail have no direct antibacterial or antiviral effect, they do provide antimicrobial protection through stimulation of the host immune function. This includes increased production of interferons and stimulation of macrophage activity. In addition, Turkey Tail has shown the above-mentioned ability to increase action and maturation of DCs and T-cells, leading to an increased cellular immune response to attack microorganisms (Hobbs, 2004).

Active Components

Beta glucans
Proteanated polysaccharides such as:
      PSP (an isolated polysaccharopeptide)
      PSK beta (1,4)-D glucan protein
Ergosterol derivatives (a form of Vitamin D2)

Side Effects

Turkey Tail, like many medicinal mushrooms, is remarkable for the lack of negative side effects experienced by its users in clinical trials and more than thirty years of testing and clinical use. A few people using PSK or PSP on a daily basis have reported darkening of the fingernails. Coughs have been reported rarely.

Collection and Preservation

Turkey Tail is collected during active growth in the late summer or fall of the year. The fruiting bodies often grow in large numbers on a single log and lend themselves to collection en masse. Though the mushrooms are persistent and can be found throughout the year, do not collect old or dead mushrooms, but only those with a fresh, pure-white pore surface. The flexible clusters of mushrooms are easily stripped off wood by pulling them up or to the side of the log. It is much more difficult to cut the mushrooms off the wood, even with the sharpest knife. Often, bits of the bark or moss will adhere to the base of the mushrooms. These are easily removed by hand or, more cleanly, with a pair of sharp scissors back at home.

I lay out the cleaned Turkey Tails on a screen in the warm attic of my barn or, in smaller quantities, in an electric dehydrator. Due to their thin flesh, they quickly dry into crisp, tough chips that can easily be stored in plastic freezer bags. At times, as the mushrooms mature, tiny larvae will begin to tunnel through the base of the brackets, as evidenced by the telltale bits chewed off at the base of the caps. It you are concerned that you might be harboring a crop of these larvae, place the freezer bag with your dried Turkey Tails in the freezer overnight.

Preparation and Use

The best way to extract the greatest proportion of useful compounds from dried or fresh Turkey Tails at home is by simmering them in water. I have attempted to powder dried Turkey Tail in a food processor and blender *before cooking* and found this to be an exercise in frustration and a significant strain on my aging food processor.

To use Turkey Tails, add enough cold water to the fresh or dried mushrooms to cover them well and bring them to a boil. After a few minutes, use a slotted spoon to transfer the softened mushrooms and a bit of the cooking water into the bowl of a food processor fitted with a metal blade. Pulse the material until it is reduced to coarse slurry, adding more water as needed. Transfer the slurry back into the pan containing the remaining cooking liquid and continue to simmer it over low heat for up to an hour. Add more water as needed. The idea is to keep the mixture the consistency of a soup, not oatmeal. Strain the mix through a metal strainer; if you have cheesecloth, line the strainer with several layers of it, and after the liquid drains, squeeze out any remaining liquid. The mushroom bits can then be discarded. If the broth is not used immediately, it can be put in a glass container and refrigerated for up to a week. The broth can be used in many ways.

I use it as a base for soups or add it to soups, stews, or sauces. The broth can also be frozen in ice-cube trays for both storage and portioning. Once solid, the cubes store well in freezer bags.

Turkey Tail can also be made into a tincture by double extraction (see directions on page 125) to concentrate the active components or added to a mixed tincture. In this species, the tincturing acts mostly to preserve the blend, and the alcohol in the mix tends to precipitate out some of the polysaccharides, so be sure to shake up the tincture before each use to distribute the components.

PSK is becoming more readily available as a dietary supplement in the United States. One source of PSP and PSK that has been active for a number of years is JHS Natural Products in Eugene, Oregon. The most common dosage in clinical trials and for daily use in clinical settings is five hundred milligrams to one gram three times daily.

Chapter 10

Oyster Mushroom *(Pleurotus ostreatus* and *P. populinus)*

Common names: Oyster Mushroom, Hiratake or Tomogitake (Japan) (PHOTOGRAPHS ON PAGES 72–73)

New England is packed with sugar maples. Every rural roadside and farmhouse field seems dotted with mature specimens of this handsome tree that so defines the region's heritage. With their mature trunks often exceeding two feet in diameter, and their canopy providing much-needed shade on a hot summer day, maples are stout reminders of our history as rural dwellers. In the late winter, the rising sap, tapped, collected, and boiled down to the consistency of 30-weight motor oil, becomes the sweetener that defines a New England breakfast, maple syrup.

Though I can almost taste buttery waffles with drizzles of syrup as I write this, I am more interested in the sugar maples of autumn, when these over-mature matrons become host to a spectacular display of the Oyster Mushroom. An older maple commonly begins to decline when the central leader begins to die back. This dying or dead wood becomes food for the rapacious Oyster Mushroom, hungry for the heartwood cellulose and lignins that make up its main food source. Oysters are so successful at using cellulose for food that you can purchase kits to grow this mushroom on a roll of toilet paper! I do not recommend growing medicinal mushrooms on toilet paper, but I use the example to illustrate the vigor of this hungry wood-decomposer. In late fall, I have come upon dead or dying sugar maples fruiting with at least seventy-five pounds of beautiful Oyster Mushrooms (see photo on p. 72).

Oysters are one of the edible mushrooms I refer to as season extenders, fruiting initially after the first frosts of mid-autumn and continuing well into November on the northern New England coast. Given this cycle, Oyster Mushrooms are quite frost-hardy, but occasionally a cluster will get caught by a hard freeze. These frozen masses can be collected later, though they will never be top-quality.

Oyster Mushrooms also grace our forests and fill our collecting baskets at the opposite end of the growing season. In the cool, rainy weather of late May and June, Oyster Mushrooms fruit heavily on the dead branches and trunks of the poplar tree, *Populus tremuloides,* known as the quaking aspen and, in New England, simply as poplar or popple. Oyster Mushrooms also grow on other, closely related species of poplars and are common on big-tooth aspen and balsam poplar in more northern regions and at higher elevations. In cool, wet summers, the mushrooms continue to fruit well into July, especially in more northern and higher-elevation regions.

Description

The Oyster Mushroom produces a firm, fleshy fruiting body with a broad cap ranging in color from cream white to gray to tan, sometimes with lilac overtones. The clusters of mushrooms grow shelflike in overlapping clusters directly from the wood or, at times, with a short, hairy lateral stalk. When the mushroom fruits on the upper surface of a log lying on the forest floor, it will look almost funnel-shaped. The caps are two to five inches broad and occasionally larger, shaped like a scallop shell to a semicircle, convex when young and flattening out with age. The margin of the cap will often become wavy or lobed at maturity. The gills are pure white, closely spaced, and decurrent (running down the stalk, if present), and become yellowed with age. The stalk is quite firm and short, generally strongly off-center, and almost furry with mycelia. The spore print is white to pale lilac-gray.

Occurrence and Habitat

Oyster Mushrooms often grow as a tightly packed cluster of overlapping and shelving caps, though they can appear as a single or a small cluster of caps. They are typically found on the stumps of cut trees, downed logs, and the standing timber of dead or dying trees. On a large tree, the mushrooms can grow on a dead limb or dying portion of an otherwise quite healthy tree.

Older mushroom field guides include *P. populinus* as a spring-fruiting form of the standard Oyster Mushroom, *P. ostreatus*, but it has been recently recognized as a separate species. The spring Oysters are prevalent in bottomland woods or the low-lying woods surrounding water. In the dark browns and spring greens of the early June forest, the pale, creamy mushrooms shine like a beacon against the dark tree trunks and are easily spotted from up to forty yards away. The mushrooms will fruit from near ground level and up thirty to forty feet on the upper trunk of the tree. A long forked stick can be quite effective at prying the out-of-reach clusters off the tree, and harvesting high-growing mushrooms is a good way to improve your hand-eye coordination as you attempt to catch the falling clusters before they hit the ground.

Though the Oyster Mushroom can be found from spring through early winter, we rarely see it after the late spring flush until October, when it is found most abundantly on sugar maple and, with less enthusiasm, on other hardwood species. On large, weakened maple trees it can produce dozens of large fruiting clusters with a combined weight in excess of fifty pounds for several years running before exhausting the available food source.

Oyster Mushrooms can be found worldwide growing and fruiting on a wide assortment of trees. In my native New Mexico and throughout the Southwest, I see *P. ostreatus* fruiting most heavily on the stately old cottonwoods that line the watercourses. Huge clusters of Oyster Mushrooms can be picked from the thick trunks of these trees following the fall rains and occasionally in the spring. In the higher elevations of the Southwest, as in New England, *P. populinus* can be found in the spring and early summer growing on the trembling aspen, a common fire-successional tree that rapidly fills the empty spaces left by forest fires above nine thousand feet.

Ecological Information

The Oyster Mushroom is an aggressive saprobe, rapidly colonizing its host tree and causing significant rot. Along with other wood-rotting fungi, it plays a vital role in breaking down dead-wood waste and recycling the nutrients bound up in the tissue. Though we often refer to Oyster Mushrooms as fruiting on trees, they are also common on logs and branches on the forest floor, where they are more prone to attack by slugs, which love them at least as much as we do. Different species and varieties of Oyster Mushrooms grow commonly in almost every climate able to support tree growth. They have been domesticated for many years in a number of countries and can be easily cultivated at home on hardwood logs. Mushrooms grown on sawdust "logs," or on other materials such as straw and other agricultural waste, are available in stores year-round.

Edibility

The Oyster Mushroom is edible and highly esteemed by many. The tough stem is usually removed, if present, and the mushroom is generally at its best for eating when collected young. Be aware that many insects love Oyster Mushrooms, so examine your find for beetles, grubs, and other insects, and use it up quickly lest others use it first. I have found that the varieties that fruit late in the season escape most insect predation, a small reward for cold-weather collecting.

The Oyster Mushroom has a high protein content, varying from 15 to 40 percent dry weight, depending on the protein content of the substrate; several B vitamins; and all the essential amino acids except tryptophan. In many tropical countries, protein is the limiting nutrient in a diet rich in carbohydrates, and the result is often malnourished children and adults. The many species and varieties of Oyster Mushrooms are easy to grow and capable of turning agricultural waste into relatively high-protein food for rural populations. This has led to efforts to teach farmers the skills needed to cultivate this valuable protein source using materials such as banana leaves or rice straw as a substrate.

Look-alikes

The Angel Wing, *Pleurocybella porrigens*, is a small, thin Oysterlike mushroom that grows on dead softwood logs. Often it fruits on the ground on partially buried wood. In Japan, fourteen poisoning deaths were attributed to this mushroom in 2004. All the victims were older (fifty-nine to seventy-five) and had a history of chronic kidney failure. This mushroom has long been considered a safe edible, and no known poisonings have occurred in United States. The 2004 cases were the first poisonings noted worldwide.

Other Oyster Mushrooms related to *P. ostreatus* include *P. dryinus*, Veiled Oyster, which is generally a larger, thick-fleshed fruit with a distinct and often central stalk, soft white scale-like fibers on the cap, and a tendency to age or bruise yellow. Young mushrooms show a veil over the gills or attached to the stalk or the edge of the cap. It is edible, though somewhat tough.

The Elm Oyster, *Hypsizygus tessulatus,* fruits in the autumn on similar hardwood tree species as the Oyster Mushroom. It resembles the Oyster but with a more pronounced and more central stalk. It is also edible.

Folk or Traditional Medicinal Uses

The Oyster Mushroom is traditionally used for food.

Current Medicinal Uses

Immunomodulation (due to glucan content) and treatment of high cholesterol. The Oyster Mushroom is reportedly used in the Czech Republic as the main ingredient of a dietary supplement for treating high cholesterol (Hobbs, 1995).

Areas of Research

Antitumor activity: Several studies with mice, rats, and hamsters have shown strong tumor reduction with both the oral feeding of whole fruiting bodies and the injection of a polysaccharide fraction (Hobbs, 1995). The lectins in Oyster Mushroom have also shown antitumor effects in animal studies.

High-cholesterol treatment: The Oyster Mushroom has been shown to lower blood cholesterol in several experiments with rats and rabbits (Chorvathova et al., 1993; Lindequist et al., 2005; and Shahdat et al., 2003) in which animals were fed a diet of up to 10 percent dried fruiting bodies as part of their normal nutritional intake. Recent studies have isolated a naturally occurring form of Lovastatin, a drug approved for treating high cholesterol in this country. In another study using hamsters (Daba, 2005), a glucan fraction extracted with ethanol was shown to reduce cholesterol, though not as significantly as in hamsters fed whole, dried fruiting bodies of Oyster Mushrooms. Studies in rabbits also reported a lowering of cholesterol, and that animals fed Oyster Mushrooms also showed a reduction in the development of plaques in major arteries (Babek et al., 1998). A human clinical trial is under way exploring the lipid-reducing possibilities of Oyster Mushrooms in patients with HIV.

Active Components
Polysaccharides
> Beta-1,3-D glucan (Pleuran)
> Alpha glucans

Lectins
Peptides: Pleurostrin
Lovastatin-like compound (for reducing cholesterol)
Ergosterols (Provitamin D2)

Toxicity
There is no known toxicity resulting from the use of Oyster Mushrooms as food or dietary supplements. Oyster Mushrooms have been commonly and safely eaten in many areas of the world for generations.

Where Oyster Mushrooms are cultivated in large-scale operations, some workers exposed repeatedly to high spore concentrations can develop an allergic reaction resulting in inflammation of the lungs. This could become a problem in homes where people cultivate their own mushrooms, though the allergic response requires repeated exposures. Like most large, fleshy mushrooms, Oysters drop huge quantities of spores when mature. A large cluster left on the kitchen table overnight can release hundreds of millions of spores.

Collection, Preparation, and Use

Since Oysters combine the edibility of a great mushroom with the health-promoting properties of a strong immune stimulator, they are best used as a tasty functional food. Collect firm, fresh young mushrooms and eat a few as a taste and textural addition to a dish, or make Oyster Mushrooms your main course. The clusters are often quite easily pulled off or cut from the tree at the base of the cap. I prefer to collect and eat those mushrooms where the cap is not yet fully expanded and the margin is still slightly rolled. Older fall mushrooms can become dense and chewy and less desirable for eating fresh, though these can be dried for medicinal use or for addition to soups or stews. Older mushrooms can also be slowly stewed or braised to tenderize them.

Dried Oysters can be easily powdered in a blender or food processor and taken in capsules or added to broth or soup stock. I would recommend the dried mushrooms be cooked to increase access to the medicinal components. Using Oyster Mushrooms along with other medicinal mushrooms provides a broader range of glucans, and therefore a broader immune system response.

For use in treating high cholesterol, eat the mushrooms regularly or take powdered, dried mushrooms daily. Here the ongoing use of the mushrooms is ideal, as high cholesterol tends to be a chronic condition in the absence of diet and lifestyle change.

Chapter 11

Chaga *(Inonotus obliquus)*

Common names: Birch Clinker, False Tinder Conk, Kabanoanatake (Japan)
(PHOTOGRAPHS ON PAGE 74)

For wild-mushroomers, winter is a time to consume the stores of dried or frozen edibles laid up during the productive summer and fall mushrooming season. It is a time to look at our field guides, research new species and ideas, search the mushroom sites on the Web, and, in short, dream about the mushroom season ahead. As my friend Michaeline says, "Winter is the time to walk in the forest remembering where you found mushrooms in summers and autumns past." But while you are consuming the last of your dried Black Trumpets and carefully rationing the meager stores of frozen sautéed Chanterelles, consider that some mushroomers are still out in the woods collecting one type of fungi for their year-round use. The fungus I refer to is Chaga, *Inonotus obliquus,* also known in this country as the Birch Clinker, and in Japan as Kabanoanatake.

The name Chaga comes from Siberia, where this fungus has been revered for several centuries as a cure-all for many maladies. I do not usually refer to Chaga as a mushroom because the most visible portion of Chaga, the part collected and used, is not the Chaga's fruiting body. Rather it is a **sclerotium,** a concentration of the vegetative growth of the fungus, the hyphae, which normally do not produce spores. A sclerotium can be described as a fungal energy storage organ, much like an onion or potato, that concentrates the products of growth until the conditions are right for the production of fruiting bodies. A number of mushroom species produce fruiting bodies from underground sclerotia, including Morels, *Grifola (Polyporus) umbellatus*, and certain tropical Oyster Mushrooms. Chaga differs from most fungi by producing a sclerotium aboveground, attached to the side of the host tree, rather than underground.

Description
Chaga belongs to the woody polypore group of fungi. Its close relatives produce leathery to corky annual polypore-fruiting bodies on wood or on the ground, fruiting from buried wood. The Chaga sclerotium erupts from the trunk of a living tree, usually a birch, at the site of a wound or where a branch has broken off the

tree. Chaga can occur anywhere from ground level up, and occasionally at thirty feet or higher on the trunk of a large tree.

The Chaga can be rounded but is usually irregularly shaped, with an outer surface made up of dense black or dark-brown material breaking into an angular crust. It looks like something that has been fused by fire and cracked on cooling; hence the common name Clinker. This is not a fungus that makes one look for the sauté pan and olive oil! Under that very hard black surface, the interior is brown to golden-brown, mottled, and has the consistency of firm cork.

The whole mass can be more than fifteen inches across and may protrude from the trunk for almost as many inches, generally becoming smaller in diameter farther from the tree. At other times the Chaga mass appears to frame the opening created by a broken branch or to line an injury to the bark. In actuality, the expanded Chaga is the result of a sclerotium slowly growing outward over several years. Often one will see bits of birch bark, and sometimes outer layers of wood, caught up in the expanding Chaga. The actual fruiting body producing the spores of the fungus is small, inconspicuous, and not often seen.

I have seen several Chaga "framing" a woodpecker's nest hole. I assume the crafty bird chose the Chaga-softened heartwood for its home. This same habit has been observed and reported upon in the western United States, where woodpeckers seek out mature Douglas fir with fruiting bodies of *Fomitopsis pinicola*, the Red-belted Polypore, and dig out a nesting cavity in the wood softened by the fungus.

Occurrence and Habitat

Chaga is a cold-loving fungus found most commonly in the boreal forests of the circumpolar north. It grows as a parasite predominantly on species of birch, though it also attacks alder, elm, and hornbeam. Only those growing on birch have been recommended and studied for medicinal use. It is most commonly found on trees in areas with a high water table and/or high humidity, such as bottomlands near bogs or on banks and slopes along lakes, streams, and rivers. It occurs frequently, if not commonly, throughout northern New England and farther north throughout much of Canada and Alaska. In southern New England, Chaga can be found only in more mountainous localities with colder climates. Chaga is slow-growing and therefore most easily found on mature trees, especially paper and yellow birch. Because gray birch is relatively short-lived, Chaga is less frequently found on this species. Chaga also grows on black or sweet birch in more southerly locations. Present throughout the year, it is traditionally gathered in the winter, perhaps because it is more visible when leaves are off the trees or the wet bottomlands are frozen solid for walking. A mature Chaga sclerotium with a six-inch diameter is estimated to be six to eight years old. In Siberia, the most highly prized Chaga grows on black birch.

Ecological Information

Chaga is a parasite. I have seen it growing on a mature tree for many years, and such trees often have significant deformities in the area of infection. The bark and outer layers of the heartwood become incorporated into the outer layer of the growing Chaga, leaving a depression and scar on the tree if the sclerotium is removed or dies. It has been my observation that if the tree dies, the Chaga sclerotium also dies within the same year. I do not know if this is due to the over-competition of other fungi, such as *Fomes fomentarius* and *Piptoporus betulinus,* or if Chaga is unable to continue growth as a pure saprobe. At times, trees seem to "throw off" the infection, though they continue to carry a distinctive scar. I regularly see yellow birch, in particular, with several scars where a Chaga had grown in the past. Such trees often have one or more active Chaga as well. On other trees, especially paper or gray birch, a Chaga "infection" commonly leads to the death of the tree. Growth of the Chaga mycelium in the heartwood of the tree weakens the wood, and I frequently come upon recently dead birches in the forest where the wind has snapped the trunk cleanly off at the site of a Chaga growth.

Edibility

Chaga is not considered edible in the sense that a Morel or Chanterelle is. Its woody consistency makes it too dense; think of eating a wine cork. It is well suited to grinding for a tea or tincture.

Toxicity

There is no evidence that Chaga is toxic or that the hot-water decoction is not well tolerated.

Folk or Traditional Medicinal Uses

Chaga has been used primarily in Russia and other Baltic countries for at least three hundred years as a general tonic and a treatment for cancers, including breast, pulmonary, skin, rectal, and stomach, as well as for other gastric ailments. It has also been used to address liver or heart disease and worms. Traditionally, chunks of the sclerotium, with the black outer rind removed, were boiled and the decoction drunk as a tea. This tea was also used for enemas in treating colon cancers and other lower-bowel complaints. The "grounds" that remained after making tea were mashed into a poultice and used to promote skin healing and as an anti-bacterial (Stamets, 2002).

Chaga was also considered an internal cleansing agent and has been used for pain control. In 1955, following some years of research and testing, Chaga was approved for the treatment of cancers by the Medical Academy of Science in Moscow (Hobbs, 1995). After noticing that the residents of Kamchatka, an area in northeastern Russia, showed no incidence of stomach cancer, scientists made an effort to determine the cause. They concluded that the regular consumption of Chaga tea from an early age was the contributing factor (Chang, 2000). Chaga has also been used traditionally for general pain relief and to address inflammation.

According to Christopher Hobbs (1995), the Khanty people, native to parts of western Siberia, continue to use Chaga tea in their traditional way to treat tuberculosis, stomachache, and diseases of the stomach, liver, and heart. It is also used as a general cleansing agent and to treat intestinal worms.

Though the native peoples of North America used Chaga, our knowledge of their methods is certainly incomplete.

Fungal Firestarters

One of the common names for *Inonotus obliquus* is False Tinder Conk, alluding to the use of this mushroom for starting fires. I first learned this from several "primitive-skills practitioners" at Maine Organic Farmers and Gardeners Association's annual Common Ground Country Fair, where I was giving out samples of Chaga chai (tea). They were as surprised at the use of Chaga as a tea as I was of its use as a firestarter, and I can't help thinking that we each harbored judgments about the manner in which the other "wasted" a favorite fungus.

Prior to the invention of the friction match in 1826, flint and steel were used to start fires. Earlier, a variety of simple friction devices were used to produce the 800 degrees Fahrenheit needed to ignite fine tinder. Tinder had to have the capacity to catch the spark easily and keep the newly created ember alive until it could be transferred to more substantial fuel. Finely shredded or powdered Chaga is known as excellent tinder for this use. The corky inner tissue of whole, dried Chaga can be set aglow to produce an ember that will continue to smolder as it is carried from place to place.

Another highly regarded mushroom tinder, *Fomes fomentarius*, or Amadou, is discussed on pages 120 and 122.

Current Medicinal Uses

A preparation of Chaga licensed and brought to market in the 1960s by Russian scientists under the name Befungin is still available and widely used. It is recommended for use in Russia as a treatment or adjuvant treatment for several forms of cancer, especially of the gut, genitals, and breast. As with most immunomodulating mushrooms, the polysaccharide components stimulate the body's immune system to activate macrophages and T-cells and produce interferons, interleukins, and TNF.

In Russia, Chaga is a common treatment for psoriasis. Lotions and balms made with Chaga are used there to treat arterial and joint disease and in the healing of wounds (Gorbunove et al., 2005). Many preparations and extracts are available as dietary supplements to improve the functioning of the immune system, as a protection from infection, and as a general tonic.

Areas of Research

Antitumor: Studies of cancerous mice using a water- and ethanol-based extract of "a yet-to-be delineated polysaccharide component" of Chaga, taken orally, have shown the extract to have significant antitumor effects (Kim et al., 2006). The basis of a fourfold increase in survival rates was through stimulation of immune components such as B-cells and macrophages in the mice rather than by direct action against the tumors.

Betulin and betulinic acid, which are found in the outer black "skin" of Chaga sclerotium, have shown promise in the treatment of the skin cancer melanoma in laboratory studies utilizing mice. It also demonstrated anticancer activity against a number of other cancer cell lines in culture studies (Eiznhamer and Xu, 2004). Cancer growth is impeded by the induction of programmed cell death (apoptosis) in tumor cells (Tang et al., 2003).

A number of distinct bioactive triterpenes have been isolated from Chaga. Among the most abundant is inotodiol, which has shown "potent" antitumor activity (Nakata et al., 2006, and Taji, 2008).

Antioxidant and free-radical scavenging: With the increased interest in the damage caused by free radicals in the body and their implications for aging and the induction of cancers, the fact that Chaga extracts show marked antioxidant potential has garnered a great deal of attention.

The melanin component, which is present in higher concentrations in the dark rind of Chaga, has been shown to have significant antioxidative action

(Babitskaya et al., 2002). This activity helps protect the genetic material of the cells from the mutation caused by reactive oxidation. Another study (Nakata et al., 2006) sought to differentiate between the antioxidant capacity of the black outer rind and the brown interior and noted that while both components showed very high antioxidative capacity, the activity from the black rind was due to small phenolic compounds extracted with alcohol, while a hot-water decoction of the interior flesh had the highest antioxidant potential.

Cultures of Chaga mycelia grown in the presence of hydrogen peroxide (a cause of oxidative stress in cells) were stimulated to produce higher concentrations of melanin and other antioxidant compounds (Zheng et al., 2008).

A water-soluble extract of Chaga has shown antioxidant effects in cell culture trials. Many scientists believe that oxidative nuclear DNA damage over the human life span strongly contributes to age-related degeneration and the development of cancers (Park et al., 2004).

The triterpene extract as well as a polyphenol extract of Chaga showed antioxidant activity and the ability to protect cells from oxidative stress (Yong et al., 2005).

Anti-inflammatory: Ethanol extracts of Chaga have shown marked, dose-dependent ability to inhibit the production of the chemical mediators of inflammation, leading to a reduction in the body's inflammatory response (Kim et al., 2007).

An alcohol extract of Chaga, likely triterpenes, has demonstrated anti-inflammatory and pain-relieving properties in animal tests (Park et al., 2005). This supports the traditional uses of this fungus to address pain and inflammation.

Anti-hyperglycemic: Diabetic rats fed a diet including 5 percent Chaga or fermented Chaga powder showed a considerable increase in chemical markers, indicating reduced blood-sugar levels and increased insulin sensitivity (Jae-Young et al., 2005).

Other uses: There is also evidence to support the use of betulinic acid for its antimicrobial properties and betulinic acid derivatives to treat HIV. The betulin in Chaga is taken from the birch host and concentrated up to 30 percent in the outer skin of the sclerotium. Many betulinic acid compounds are sold as dietary supplements and recommended by herbalist practitioners.

Active Components
Triterpenes (lanostanoid-type and others)
Melanin complex

Heteropolysaccharides including beta glucans
Protein-bound polysaccharide (xylogalactoglucose)
Inositols (B vitamins)
Inotodiol
Ergosterols (Provitamin D) and other sterols
Betulin and betulinic acid (concentrated from birch bark)

Collection and Preservation

The sclerotium of the Chaga is quite suitable for collection in the winter, a time when we often need a reason to leave a warm chair for the great outdoors. Searching for Chaga keeps me aware of the trunks of trees, and I have been amazed at how many woodpecker holes, owls' nests, and other tree-hollow homes I see. It is important to note that I would not recommend winter for collecting medicinal fungi other than Chaga. The best time for collecting other species is when the fruiting bodies are actively growing or approaching maturity.

Chaga is best collected using a hatchet or a broad chisel and a hammer to pry off the growth without unnecessary damage to the growing tree. Since *Inonotus obliquus* is a parasite, it might benefit the tree to remove the sclerotium, though this would not end the colonization of the tree by the fungus.

You will need to address your frustration at having to pass up those Chaga growing high above your head. I have found myself shinning up some trees better left to the skills of an active twelve-year-old. At times it is easy to break off the Chaga from below with a stick without causing any damage to the tree or yourself. It might be advisable to wear a hard hat if you try this, as you will be dislodging several pounds of dense material from directly overhead.

Preparation and Use

Chaga has been prepared and is still available commercially (in Ukraine and Russia) as a tea, syrup, extract, suppository, tablet, aerosol, and injection (Hobbs, 1995). Several companies market liquid extracts, and Chaga can be found as an ingredient in many herbal preparations.

Chaga is most commonly prepared as a hot tea (decoction) made from the ground sclerotium. Traditionally, in Russia, only the inner golden or light-brown part is used. The fresh or dried Chaga is broken into chunks, boiled for a long time, and then drunk hot or cold. Since we now know that valuable betulin and betulinic acid and other (alcohol-extracted) compounds are found in the black outer skin, that part should be used as well. Made either way, the tea is a refreshing beverage, hot or cold. A review of the literature shows different recommendations for preparing a hot-water decoction of Chaga. While many recommend boiling, others suggest a long (up to forty-eight hours) steeping with warm water. One study of the Chaga's antitumor activity showed that the active anticancer components are increased in the tea by boiling a decoction and virtually absent in the non-boiled tea. Since a hot-water extraction is necessary to access the polysaccharides that stimulate host immune response, I would not recommend the warm-water–steeping method.

To Prepare Chaga Tea

Use 2 to 4 tablespoons of Chaga (ground or in as small pieces as possible) to 2 quarts of water. Heat to boiling and allow to gently simmer for at least 20 minutes. (Longer simmering results in a more bitter tea but also increases terpene levels.) The grounds can be reused once. Drink one small cup daily for general system maintenance, or two or three cups a day for immune-system boosting or to address specific complaints. Chaga decoctions make a great base for your daily coffee, and coffee products made with Chaga are on the market. The author prepares and is marketing Chaga Chai made with Maine Chaga and organic spices.

A tincture or double-extraction tincture (page 125) is most effective in concentrating the triterpene components along with the polysaccharides. Tinctures can be used daily in water, juice, or tea as an immune-booster tonic. The anti-inflammatory properties help in avoiding respiratory ailments and gastrointestinal-related disorders or other inflammation-related issues.

Skin-care products containing Chaga have long been made and sold in Eastern Europe and are now beginning to appear in the United States.

Chapter 12

Lion's Mane *(Hericium erinaceus)* and Comb Tooth
(H. coralloides, H. americanum [ramosum])

Common names: Comb Tooth, Bear's Head Hydnum, Lion's Mane, Pom-Pom, Monkey Head, Yamabushitake, Houtou (PHOTOGRAPHS ON PAGES 75–76)

I feel an almost visceral jolt at the sudden sight of a great edible or medicinal mushroom, seen gestalt-like as pure form from a distance. Sometimes the mushroom emerges from the obscuring background of leaves and twigs like a partridge frozen on a nest under a snag. Your brain begins to question the pattern it sees, and then, *snap*, you are able to see the whole, as if it had instantly materialized. This happens to those of us who seek the Black Trumpet, that delicious, delicate, impossibly well-hidden member of the Chanterelle family. The mind embraces the form enough to see one, and, if you stop to really look, an entire small village of Trumpets emerges from the duff.

For those who seek the Lion's Mane or the similar Comb Tooth, finding these mushrooms provides a comparable jolt. Picture a clean, white mass of mushroom growing from the dark-gray bark of a dead standing beech tree in the dark understory of a mixed beech and hemlock woods. The pure white mushroom contrasts with the gloom of the background like a gold doubloon lying on a black-sand beach. It captures your attention in a split second.

The Comb Tooth grabbed the attention of the scientific and healing community with the discovery of erinacine E, described as a potent stimulator of nerve growth factor synthesis. Research suggested that these nerve growth factors (NGF) could play a role in treating many disorders of the nervous system, including Alzheimer's disease and other forms of dementia.

I get ahead of myself. The genus *Hericium* in New England is represented by three species. *H. erinaceus,* known as the Lion's Mane, Bear's Head, or Pom-Pom, is the best-known member of the genus. Most of the medicinal research done on *Hericium* has been carried out with this species, and it is also the easiest of the three to identify. *H. erinaceus* is rare in the north and becomes more common the farther south one travels from New England in the eastern half of the United States. The other two species, *H. americanum* and *H. coralloides,* are instantly recognizable as members of this genus, but depending on the book you consult, you might call them one of several confusing and overlapping names. Fortunately, the confusion over names need not get in the way of enjoying these mushrooms as food or appreciating their medicinal attributes. All three are excellent and safe edibles, especially when collected and cooked while young and white. There is evidence that they share many of the same medicinal components, and erinacine E has been isolated from both *H. erinaceus and H. coralloides.*

Description

The fruiting bodies of both *H. americanum* and *H. coralloides* rise directly attached to wood, without an obvious stem, and mature to a roughly globose to irregular shape ranging from four inches to a foot in diameter. Each mushroom is pure white and darkens with age to reddish-brown and brown, especially at the tips. Young fruiting bodies are at times pink to almost salmon (page 76 photo).

Each has a central base that immediately branches out, ending in clusters of short icicle teeth. In *H. coralloides,* the teeth on a mature mushroom measure less than a half-inch long; in *H. americanum,* the teeth are longer, generally from one-half inch to an inch. *H. coralloides* branches more and has a spread-out, diffuse appearance. *H. americanum* is often more dense, with less branching, and retains the look of a compact mass on the side of a tree or log. The spines of each species droop in graceful falls, and it is along the exterior surface of these spines that the white spores mature and are released.

H. erinaceus differs from the two other species in that the base does not branch and it possesses longer teeth. The long, pendulous icicle teeth arise from a simple, unbranched, tough central stalk and can be up to six centimeters long. The whole fruiting body can be more than a foot in diameter and is generally solitary on the stumps or logs of trees. Until recently, *H. coralloides* was known as *H. ramosum,* and many older field guides refer to it as such. Those *Hericium* with longer teeth were earlier known as *H. coralloides* but are now known as *H. americanum.* You are in good company if this confuses you, as most experienced mushroomers have difficulty with the assigned names.

Occurrence and Habitat

Look for *Hericiums* following periods of wet weather as the early fall chill comes with the night air. In a dry year, dead standing trees may not fruit, but logs and branches lying on the forest floor will still produce. I find them earliest on beech and, later, maple and birch, especially white birch. Fruiting can continue through autumn.

All three species favor hardwoods. In New England, *H. americanum* and *H. coralloides* prefer beech, maple, and birch. *H. americanum* is commonly found on the dead standing or downed logs of beech and occasionally at the site of an injury on a living tree. *H. coralloides* is more prone to fruit on logs lying on the ground, perhaps because the higher humidity at ground level is more conducive to growth. Look for them as solitary growths or, more commonly, as several clusters growing along the surface of a log or tree. On the forest floor, they emerge on the lower sides and even the underside of a log that is raised above the forest floor. The mushrooms emerge from ground level to more than twenty feet up on the trunk of a larger tree. When you find a tree producing Comb Tooth, make note of the location and seek it out the following year under similar weather conditions. It will likely fruit again at about the same time.

H. erinaceus is often found growing on oak, beech, or maple and is not typically found on birch.

Ecological Information

The *Hericiums* are primarily saprobes and weak parasites, invading a living tree at the site of a wound and colonizing the dead heartwood. They can also live on and break down dead wood and appear to be quite aggressive at degrading wood. Within a very few years from the onset of fruiting, a log a foot in diameter is already broken down to the point that it no longer produces mushrooms.

Edibility

Unlike many groups of fungi, where you must know the species to determine edibility, it really doesn't matter which species in the genus *Hericium* you have. All are very good edibles and have no history of causing difficulties when consumed. *Hericium* are best when eaten young, tender, and pure white. As they age, becoming cream-colored or with brown teeth, they, like many fleshy mushrooms, are prone to be colonized by mold or bacteria that could render them toxic. We would not consider eating hamburger left out for a couple of days; the same consideration should be used for mushrooms. Eat them when they are firm, fresh, and show no signs of decay. *Hericium* have the reputation for cooking up with a slight taste of seafood—lobster, some say. They are a welcome addition to a milk- or cream-based chowder.

Toxicity

People eating this mushroom or using it as a dietary supplement have reported no problems.

Look-alikes

As already mentioned, all species in the genus *Hericium* found growing in the
United States are good edibles. The species may be difficult to tell apart within the
genus but have few, if any, real look-alikes. The species of *Hericium* that include *H.
coralloides* and *H. americanum* (as well as *H. ramosum* and *H. laciniatum)* are similar in
appearance and somewhat variable. The medicinally better-known *H. erinaceus* is
found occasionally in New England but is more common farther south and even
into the tropics.

Note: Though I recommend without hesitation that the related forms of *Hericium*
can be lumped together in terms of edibility, I am less comfortable making a
similar statement regarding their medicinal values, though I am inclined to do so.
Most research into the medicinal properties of *Hericium* has been carried out using
H. erinaceus, but several studies comparing the polysaccharide components of *H.
coralloides* and *H. laciniatum* with *H. erinaceus* have shown that, while there are some
differences in the sugar makeup of the polysaccharides, their antitumor effect in
studies using mice was very similar, as was the reported stimulation in the production of immune factors such as T-cells and macrophages (Wang et al., 2001). In
addition, the erinacine isolated from *H. erinaceus* and seen as a nerve growth stimulator has also been isolated from *H. ramosum* and *H. coralloides* (Saito et al., 1998).
These two findings lead me to suggest that all Northeastern *Hericium* can be used
as a health-promoting dietary supplement with similar benefits. No analysis of the
medical components of *H. americanum* has been published.

Folk or Traditional Medicinal Uses

Hericium species have been used as food in a number of areas around the globe for
many years, most notably in China and Japan. Until recently, the medicinal use of
these mushrooms has been more limited, and this may be due primarily to the relative rarity of the fruiting bodies in the wild. *Hericium* is not common in most regions.
As artificial cultivation of this wood-degrader has improved over the past twenty
years, the mushrooms are more available year-round for research and use.

Current Medicinal Uses

Powdered fruiting bodies and mycelium are sold by a number of sources as dietary
supplements, generally as capsules of dried mycelium, and recommended for use
as immune stimulants and for improved brain function. At this time in the United
States, the FDA has approved no medical uses for this mushroom.

Areas of Research

Nerve growth factor stimulant: The most exciting aspect of the medicinal value of *Hericium* has been the discovery and study of erinacines that show the ability to stimulate the production of nerve growth factor (NGF) in animal trials and hold promise as possible therapeutic agents in the treatment of Alzheimer's disease and other neurodegenerative disorders (Yamada et al., 1997). The erinacines are diterpenoid compounds that are potent stimulators of the production of NGF and have been shown to increase some neurotransmitter levels and to increase levels of NGF in the brains of experimental rats given doses of erinacines into the stomach (Shimbo, Kawagishi, and Yokogoshi, 2005). However, a study using human brain astrocytoma cells (Koichiro et al., 2008) showed that while a methanol extract of *H. erinaceus* powder stimulated an increase in NGF, the application of purified erinacines did not. This leaves in question the exact mechanism of NGF stimulation by this mushroom in human brain cell lines, but evidence shows repeatedly that *Hericium* is an effective NGF stimulator.

A recent human clinical study was carried out in Japan with a group of men and women, age fifty to eighty, diagnosed with mild cognitive impairment and treated with *H. erinaceus* fruiting body powder given orally. This double-blind, placebo-controlled study showed that the treatment group subjects had significant improvement in cognitive function at eight, twelve, and sixteen weeks, and that the improvement did not last beyond four weeks after the dose was discontinued. The test subjects were given one gram of dry powder three times per day (Mori et al., 2008). All fourteen test subjects showed improved cognitive functioning at sixteen weeks as compared to five of fifteen placebo subjects.

Antitumor and immunomodulatory: Studies utilizing hot-water extracts of *Hericium* species have demonstrated effects on a number of components of immune functioning, including:

- Increased activity of macrophages and the release of nitric oxide by rat peritoneal macrophages, as well as an indication that this was due to the water-extract enhancement of the expression of the genes for nitric oxide production (Son et al., 2006)
- Indirect activation of NK cells as evidenced by an increase in interleukin-12 and interferon following treatment with a hot-water extract of Hericium used with mouse splenocytes grown out with Yac-1 lymphoma cells (Yim et al., 2007)

- Polysaccharides extracted from culture broth of *H. coralloides* and *H. erinaceus* were shown to increase the levels of T-cells and macrophages and to be active against lung cancer tumors in mice (Wang et al., 2001). Another study by the same author showed that the **antimutagenic** (enhancing the resistance of cells to become cancerous in the presence of cancer-causing agents) action of the extract from the fruiting body was greater than that of the extract from cultivated mycelium, and that an ethanol extract was better than a water extract for cancer protection in this species (Wang et al., 2001).

Active Components
Beta-D glucans
Additional bioactive and antitumor polysaccharides
Diterpinoids such as erinacines and related cyathanes (Kenmoku, 2002)
Ergosterols; Vitamin D2

Collection, Preparation, and Use
Collect *Hericium* species when they are fresh, firm, and pure white. In wet weather they can become quite waterlogged, and in such cases they need to be cooked or dried quickly to avoid spoilage. As they age, the spines become cream-to-yellow and then brown, an indication of an over-mature specimen, and flavor and texture are not as good as in a young mushroom. Consider eating the young, prime specimens and preserving any that are older but still without signs of spoilage.

As a functional food, *Hericium* is great in a stirfry, sautéed with pasta sauce, or added to soups. The stem base of *H. erinaceus* can become quite tough and may require long, slow cooking, so it might be best saved for drying.

For preparation and preservation for use as a dietary supplement for immune-system or nervous-system support, dry the fruiting body and powder it for use in capsules or added to soups and broths. For therapeutic use, use one to two grams a day or as recommended by your health-care provider. Alternatively, this is a very good mushroom to prepare in a double-extraction tincture (page 125), as research has shown that the ethanol extract contains the active nerve stimulators.

Chapter 13

Birch Polypore *(Piptoporus betulinus)*

Common names: Birch Conk, Kanbatake (Japan) (PHOTOGRAPHS ON PAGE 77)

As the overnight temperatures drop and morning walks call for a fleece covering, I begin to look for the first white knobs to emerge from the bark of the white and gray birch and announce the end of summer and the start of the Birch Polypores. By mid-September in a wet year, Birch Polypores will march up the sides of many birches, making them the most common fruiting polypore in many areas of the forest. Asked if these striking displays are edible, my answer is an equivocal "Yes, when they are young, and if you like the texture of pencil erasers."

Description

The Birch Polypore grows laterally off the trunk or side branch of a birch from a short, stout stem and occasionally along a downed log. The cap is one to ten inches wide (generally two to five inches) and semicircular to kidney- to fan-shaped as it ages. The cap top is creamy white to tan, becoming brown to dark, smoky brown, and convex with a smooth surface. The pure white flesh, initially soft and resilient, quickly takes on the consistency of a pencil eraser and then becomes corky, a half-inch to one-and-a-half inches thick. The margin of the cap is, at times, wavy in maturity and deeply enrolled, making the pore surface significantly depressed. The stalk, when present, is lateral, short, and thick, and colored like the cap. The pore surface starts out cream-white, becoming yellowish to pale tan, especially where bruised; the pores minute, three to five per millimeter, and rounded to angular. The spore print is white.

Occurrence and Habitat

The most common fungal tag-along on birch trees, this conk is abundant in the fall, actively growing from September through to hard frost. The fruiting bodies are annual, meaning that they produce only one layer of pores, but the dead conks remain on the trunks of trees through the winter. At times they are solitary on a trunk or the side branch of a birch, but, more commonly, numerous conks march up the trunk or along larger side branches (lower right photo on page 77). *Piptoporus* rapidly colonizes a dead or dying birch, and it is not unusual to find a tree

with several dozen polypores ranging from ground level to the top of all significant branches. It also frequently fruits on fallen logs.

Ecological Information

This vigorous saprobe plays a vital role in rapidly degrading the wood of birches. It
is rare to see this mushroom fruiting on the same tree for more than two consecu-
tive years, as the wood is quickly degraded and the tree falls to the forest floor. At
times, *Piptoporus* will share trunk space on a dead or dying birch with *Fomes fomentarius, Phellinus igniarius,* or other wood-degrading fungi. Because the bark of the
birch is watertight, the dead wood retains a high moisture content, making it ideal
for mycelial colonization by hungry fungal invaders.

Edibility

The Birch Polypore is reportedly edible when young, but expect it to be tough and
somewhat bitter (due to those valuable triterpenes). Fortunately, Birch Polypore
fruits at a seasonal time when the woods are generally full of more desirable
edibles. Keep the Birch Polypore for health use and seek Chanterelles and Porcini
for the table.

Look-alikes

Few fungi resembling Birch Polypore grow on birch. A small *Ganoderma applanatum,* Artist's Conk, might be found on birch (and would have similar medicinal
uses). Birch Polypore's depressed pore surface and thick, enrolled margin set it
apart from the Artist's Conk, as does its annual growth form.

Folk or Traditional Medicinal Uses

Historically, the Birch Polypore has been shredded and used as tinder for starting
fires. The dried conks were also used as an abrasive material for putting a fine finish
on razors, for which reason it was also called the razor strop fungus during Victorian
times. Medicinally, the dried, shredded conk was used to stop bleeding (Stamets, 2002).

Ötzi, the 5,300-year-old Iceman, whose extraordinarily well-preserved body
was found in the Alps after thawing out of a receding glacier along the Italian-
Austrian border, carried on his person two shaped pieces of *Piptoporus betulinus*
strung on leather thongs (Poder, 2005). There has been much speculation con-
cerning the role this mushroom played in the life of the Iceman, as well as that
of *Fomes fomentarius,* the other mushroom found in his leather satchel. Given
its antimicrobial properties and the evidence that the Iceman carried intestinal

parasites, perhaps *Piptoporus* was used to treat infectious processes. It could have also been used as a wound dressing to staunch bleeding and prevent infection.

The Birch Polypore has been used historically as a treatment for stomach ailments and for rectal cancers in Bohemia (Lindequest, 2005).

Current Medicinal Uses

Birch Polypore is not a commonly used medicinal species, in part because we are still identifying the best ways to use it. Several recently released products made with mixed mushroom species for immune enhancement include Birch Polypore and are readily available.

Areas of Research

Antimicrobial: Extracts from the fruiting body show broad-spectrum antibiotic effects (Smith et al., 2002). The fungus shows strong inhibition against *Staphylococcus aureus, Mycobacterium smegmatus, Pseudomonas aeruginosis,* and *Bacillus subtilis* (Stamets, 2002).

Nucleic acids isolated from the fruiting bodies of Birch Polypore protected mice from infection when inoculated with tick-borne encephalitis virus (Kandefer-Szerzen et al., 1979).

Tumor inhibition has been ascribed to both heteroglucans in a crude extract and also to betulinic acid, which shows promise as a treatment for melanoma (Tan et al., 2003). A polysaccharide extract showed 90 percent inhibition of growth of sarcoma 180 and Erlich solid cancers in culture tests (Ohtsuka et al., 1973).

Betulinic acid, extracted from the birch host and concentrated in the fruiting body, has demonstrated anticancer action on human melanoma cells in culture and antitumor effect in studies with mice implanted with human melanoma tumors (Pishe et al., 1995). Betulinic acid assists the induction of programmed cell death through a complex chain of actions (Tan and Pezzuto, 2003).

Anti-inflammatory: Lanostanoid-like triterpenes isolated from the fruiting body of Birch Polypore have shown significant inhibition of select pathways in the inflammatory process of the body, including prostaglandin (COX-1, COX-2, and 3-gama-HSD), a key factor in inflammation (Von Kememi Wangun, 2006).

Selected triterpenes isolated from the fruiting body have been shown to suppress edema in studies with mice (Kamo et al., 2003) and chronic dermal inflammation in studies using mice (Stamets, 2002).

Active Components
Heteroglucans
Betulin and betulinic acid (from birch host)
Triterpenes, lanostane-type
Piptamine (an antibiotic)
Ergosterols (Provitamin D2)

Collection, Preservation, Preparation, and Use
Look for fresh fruiting bodies in September and October and collect them before they show signs of decline. As they emerge from the wood, the very young, pale nubbins will contain lower concentrations of terpenes, as evidenced by their only slight bitterness, and are best left to mature before harvest. The conks are easily sliced and can be dried in a dehydrator or on screens in a warm attic or room; sun-dried fruit will increase the levels of Provitamin D2.

This mushroom can be used alone or dried and ground as one species in a mixed-species immunomodulating mixture. Given the presence of a number of triterpenes, any tincture should be made as a double extract of alcohol and hot water (see page125) to ensure that the alcohol-soluble terpenes are captured. A decoction, or tea, made from Birch Polypore will be bitter and potent. I anticipate the arrival on the market of Birch Polypore products recommended for skin care, taking advantage of both the antimicrobial and anti-inflammatory features of this fungus.

Chapter 14

Artist's Conk *(Ganoderma applanatum)*

Common name: Artist's Conk **(PHOTOGRAPHS ON PAGE 78)**

*G*anoderma applanatum, the Artist's Conk, is the poster child of the woody, durable shelf mushroom. You can be almost certain that this conk has been the comfortable recliner for a host of woodland nymphs, fairies, and sprites over the years that it has grown on the side of aged forest patriarchs. The Artist's Conk is named for the tendency of its fresh, pure-white pore surface to immediately stain brown when scratched or bruised. The surface will take a fine etching and can be used as a canvas for detailed drawings, as seen in a whimsical drawing by Maine ecologist and amateur mushroomer Kendra Bavor on page 78. Coming upon a large Artist's Conk is a memorable experience; generally, the size of the mature mushroom reflects the size and age of the tree host, so when I see one that is two feet or more across, it is invariably on a mature tree.

Description

Applanate means flat, and the Artist's Conk grows as a flattened, woody, shelflike conk on the sides of living or dead trees or downed logs. The conk is semicircular to fan-shaped, attached directly to the wood without a stem, and from two to thirty inches across, though sizes above eighteen inches are unusual. The upper surface is hard and crusty, with uneven lumps and ridges, and with a defined pattern of concentric furrows showing perennial layers of growth. The cap surface is pale grayish-brown to brown, with the outer margin usually paler. During active spore release, the upper surface can become quite rusty-brown from billions of spores adhering to the surface. The pore surface is white (to pale pinkish-brown in winter) and bruises brown when fresh. The interior flesh is brown, with the active pore layer lighter brown, and older tissue is often flecked or filled with white mycelia. Individual pores are tiny, four to six per millimeter. The spore print is brown to rusty-brown, as evidenced by a dusty layer of cinnamon-brown spores found at times on the top of the cap and surrounding surfaces.

Occurrence and Habitat

You will find the Artist's Conk growing along the trunks or branches of living or dead hardwood trees. It sometimes fruits from the roots of trees and appears at ground level as a rosette. Fruiting conks can be solitary or, more commonly, in groups, sometimes with overlapping clusters. It is perennial, adding layers of growth several times every season, and can grow for a number of years, especially on trunks of large, dense hardwood trees such as oak or maple. I frequently find smaller individuals growing on poplar trunks in moist bottomlands or along the edges of lakes, bogs, or streams. They quickly deplete the soft wood of the poplar and never grow large. This is a fairly common mushroom, especially in old-growth forests or municipal areas with mature trees.

Ecological Information
This parasitic and saprobic fungus generates white rot in the heartwood of trees it attacks. This leads to weakening of the wood and can result in blow-downs of trees at the site of the infection. Since the fungus is using only the dead heartwood as a food source, the tree can continue to live and flourish with the fungus attached for decades.

Edibility
Artist's Conk is woody and inedible.

Toxicity
This mushroom has caused no known toxic reactions. Triterpenes can render water extracts quite bitter and trigger gastrointestinal distress if taken in large amounts.

Look-alikes
Fomitopsis pinicola, the Red-belted Polypore, is generally thicker in appearance, with a marked reddish band along the upper margin and a cream-to-pale-yellow pore surface. The distinct brown interior color of the Artist's Conk distinguishes it from the Red-banded Conk with its cream-to-pale tan flesh.

Folk or Traditional Medicinal Uses
Dry fruiting bodies were burned and the smoke used as an insect repellent by native peoples in Alaska and on the west coast of America (Hobbs, 1995).

Current Medicinal Uses
Artist's Conk appears in mushroom remedies used to enhance the immune response. It is noted by Hobbs (1995) as a major ingredient in many Reishi extracts made in Taiwan, sold as immune stimulators and anti-inflammatory aids.

Areas of Research

Anti-ulcer: Polysaccharide extracts used to treat induced ulcers in rats showed stimulation of increased protective mucus secretions (Yang et al., 2005).

Antidiabetic: An in vitro study involving rats demonstrated that *G. applanatum* inhibits aldose reductase activity and strengthens glucose tolerance in diabetic rats (Jung et al., 2005). An exopolymer composed of polysaccharides with a small protein component and extracted from the mycelium of *G. applanatum* lowered plasma glucose levels in diabetic rats by 22 percent (Yang et al., 2007). Ergosterol peroxide extracted from the fruiting bodies of Artist's Conks was most effective in inhibiting the aldose reductase reaction from the eye lenses of rats (Lee et al., 2006). The aldose reductase reaction has been shown to help reduce some complications of diabetes, like vision impairment due to the buildup of pressure in the eyes.

Cholesterol-lowering: The polysaccharide-protein extract from the mycelium lowered total plasma cholesterol by 20.3 percent and triglycerides by 22.7 percent as compared to a control group of diabetic rats (Yang et al., 2007).

Antimicrobial: *G. applanatum* shows activity against a broad range of Gram-positive and Gram-negative bacteria.

Antitumor: The glucan polysaccharide components of *G. applanatum* have exhibited tumor inhibition in animal studies by several researchers (Hobbs, 1995). The exopolymer of carbohydrates and protein significantly inhibited tumor growth (39 percent more than in the control group) and raised the NK cell activity (56 percent more than controls) in mice bearing sarcoma tumors (Jeong et al., 2008). Triterpenes extracted from *G. applanatum* were shown to be effective against mouse skin-tumor promoters (Lindequest, 2005).

Immune stimulation: Glucan polysaccharides from fruiting bodies and mycelium are active immune stimulants.

Active Components

Beta glucans

Hetero-beta glucans

Triterpenes

Contains more than a hundred different terpenes, such as ganoderic acid
   and applanoxide acid (Lindequest, 2005).

Ergosterol peroxide (Provitamin D) and other sterols (Hobbs, 1995).

Ganodermadiol and other potential antibiotics

Collection, Preparation, and Use

The Artist's Conk should be collected only in the summer and fall when it is showing active growth. Though the fruits are present throughout the winter, there is no
active growth, and to all appearances the conks appear dead, with a dry, cracked
pore surface and no signs of active mycelium. The conks would have markedly
reduced medicinal value at this time.

Please consider collecting only younger, smaller fruiting bodies and leave the
stately large ones to grace the forest for the future. I try to collect this species off
aspen or poplar, where I know it is short-lived and never grows to a large size.

The collected fruiting bodies can be used fresh or dried for future use. The
dried fruiting body can be ground up and taken as a capsule or powder. The slices,
pounded or ground, can be simmered in hot water to make a somewhat bitter
decoction. The degree of bitterness is one indication of the levels of triterpenes
extracted, and increased bitterness indicates a more potent tea. This has been used
as a purgative and antibiotic as well as an immunostimulating tonic. *G. applanatum*
can also be made into a double-extraction tincture (page 125) as a good method for
concentration of the terpenes and polysaccharides.

Chapter 15

Red-belted Polypore *(Fomitopsis pinicola)*

Common names: Red-belted Conk, Red-belted Polypore, Tsugasaruno-koshikake (Japan)
(PHOTOGRAPHS ON PAGE 79)

Description

The Red-belted Polypore projects out from the side of a tree or log as a hard, woody, shelflike fruiting body. The upper surface shows concentric furrowed bands, and the outer band(s) are reddish and have a shiny, resinous surface, especially on the marginal, or newest, band. The older upper surface becomes grayish to brown. The fruiting body starts out hoof-shaped and fairly thick, becoming up to eighteen inches across and semicircular in shape. Though the expanding outer edge is thin, it rapidly thickens back to the attachment point on the host tree, making the cross section a thick, blunt wedge. The conk attaches directly to the wood without any stem; it may grow singly, or several can grow in a shelflike cluster or scattered along the trunk. The pore surface is creamy white and stains yellowish-brown when bruised or scratched. The individual pores are quite small, circular in cross-section, and three to five per millimeter. The spore print is white.

Occurrence and Habitat

The Red-belted Polypore is the most common of the large woody conks found in New England forests, especially those dominated by conifers. Found often on spruce, hemlock, or pine, it also is seen on hardwoods, especially paper or gray birch in northern New England. The perennial fruiting body can be found throughout the year. Active growth begins in the late spring and early summer and will continue through the fall, producing and releasing spores whenever the weather is wet.

Ecological Information

Fomitopsis pinicola is an aggressive saprobe, rotting the heartwood of the host. Though it occasionally infects a living host, it does not generally cause the death of a tree. It is most common on dead wood, unlike many of the other common woody polypores. Known as a brown-rot fungus, *F. pinicola* feeds on the cellulose and hemicellulose of the wood and leaves behind the dark-brown lignins that add a moisture-retaining element to the valuable humus layer of the soils. This fungus is a bane to commercial loggers as it makes infected wood weak and unusable as lumber.

Fomitopsis and Woodpeckers

When a tree is infected with a wood-rotting fungus, the structural integrity of the heartwood is lost and the wood becomes soft and spongy. Those animals which rely upon tree cavities for homes have learned that a tree with a heart-rot fungal infection is a tree already hollow, or easily made so. I have seen examples of this many times: woodpecker holes in standing trees with obvious heart rot.

This same phenomenon has been noted in western forests where logging has removed many of the mature trees normally used by cavity-nesting birds and the host of other animals, such as bats, flying squirrels, other squirrels, martens, and raccoons, that take advantage of woodpecker excavations to make their own homes. Old-growth forests contain many large dead trees, naturally creating optimum conditions for cavity creation and nesting. Extensive logging of those mature forests has led to the decline of certain cavity-nesting species, some of which, such as the Northern Spotted Owl and certain woodpeckers, are now listed as endangered. Requirements imposed by the Endangered Species Act (and political pressure from us tree-hugging nature lovers) motivated the United States Forest Service and its Canadian counterpart to devise ways to increase suitable habitat for cavity dwellers.

One technique is to inoculate both living trees and snags (dead standing trees) with wood-decaying fungi (Huss et al., 2002). Observations of nesting woodpeckers revealed that their cavity nest sites are located an average of twenty-five feet above the forest floor, so several methods of creating relatively high-altitude fungal infections have been used. The more labor-intensive method involves climbing the tree and drilling a deep hole into the heartwood, which is then filled with a plug of dowel wood colonized with the desired fungi (including *Fomitopsis pinicola*). An equally effective but less labor intensive method is to pack fungus-inoculated sawdust behind the pellets in a shotgun shell or to place a small inoculated wood dowel into an open-top, hollow rifle bullet and to blast the tree with the mushroom mycelia from the ground (Fillip et al., 2004). (Lots more fun for those boy-toy types, too—though probably not as much fun as another early experimental method: blasting off the top of large conifers with explosives.)

Follow-up studies on this creative use of fungi to restore forest habitat show successful inoculation and fungal infections well established five years later. Fruiting bodies were seen in some trees, though it was too early to know whether woodpecker cavities would follow.

Edibility

Though not toxic in any way, the Red-belted Polypore is not considered edible. You would not think of eating this tough, woody mushroom any more than you would consider eating a stick of firewood.

Look-alikes

The Red-belted Polypore can be distinguished from *Ganoderma applanatum*, the Artist's Conk, by its thicker fruiting body, creamy rather than white pore surface, and darker upper surface with the distinctive red resinous band. The Artist's Conk also prefers hardwood species in almost all cases.

Folk or Traditional Medicinal Uses

The Red-belted Polypore is used as a tonic to reduce inflammation in the gastrointestinal tract and as an immune modulator.

Current Medicinal Uses

The Red-belted Polypore is not yet widely known as a medicinal species. Studies have been limited to cell lines and lab animals. Several preparations using *F. pinicola* as one component are on the market.

Areas of Research

Antimicrobial: Scientists have recently identified a growing number of triterpenes, triterpene glycosides, and antimicrobial steroids in the fruiting body. These have shown activity against *Bacillus subtilis* (Caroline et al., 1996; and Keller, Mailklard, and Hostettmann, 1996).

Antihyperglycemic: An alkali extract made from fruiting bodies has been effective in addressing blood sugar control in induced diabetic rats and shows promise for use in this arena (Sang-Il, et al., 2008).

Anti-inflammatory: Fomitopinic acids A and B have demonstrated significant anti-inflammatory effect through inhibition of the main initiator of the inflammation cascade in the body, COX. Fomitopinic acid A has been shown to be selective for inhibition of COX-2 (Von Kamami Wagnun, HV, 2006).

Antitumor: *F. Pinicola* has been shown to be moderately tumor-inhibiting against sarcoma 180 in mice (Hobbs, 1995).

A beta-1,6 branched glucan showing strong antitumor activity in mice was isolated by Mizuno in the early 1980s (Mizuno et al., 1984).

A hot-water and an ethanol extract have both been tested using cancer cell lines. The ethanol extract showed much higher activity against human cancer cell viability rates (Choi et al., 2008).

Polysaccharides extracted from mycelial cultures showed dose-dependent inhibition in tube-cell formation in endothelial cells in culture (Cheng et al., 2008). This shows promise in inhibiting tumor-cell proliferation.

Antioxidant scavenging: The phenolic extract of *F. pinicola* showed dose-dependent antioxidant scavenging using several chemical indicators. (Choi et al., 2008).

Active Components
Ergosterol (Provitamin D)
Triterpenes and related Phenolic compounds
Fomitopinic acids A and B
Heterogalactan polysaccharides
Glucan polysaccharides showing antitumor activity
Lanostanoid steroids

Collection, Preparation, and Use
Collect only living Red-belted Polypore conks. This mushroom looks full of life even in midwinter, but harvest them during their active growing phase, from early summer through the fall.

Collecting *F. pinicola* is easy; more difficult is preparing this mushroom as a dietary supplement. This is the hardest and most fibrous of all the medicinal mushrooms, and processing it into pieces small enough to extract the medicinal components is a challenge. Fresh, young specimens are easy to cut with a sharp, heavy knife. Anything older requires a hatchet or a saw, especially if you wait until after the fruiting body has dried. I have used a band saw or hatchet to good effect, and I have read accounts of other intrepid mushroomers using a rasp, coping saw, handsaw, or the like.

The fruiting body must be pulverized to maximize the surface area to extract the most from the mushroom with a hot-water decoction. After reducing your mushroom to small pieces, place it in clean, cold water. Gently bring it to a boil and then reduce it to a simmer. Allow it to simmer for at least one hour, replacing water as needed. Use the resulting decoction as a tea alone or with other beverages. As with other decoctions, it can also be added to soups and broths. Alternatively, a double-extraction tincture (page 125) concentrates the components and utilizes the preservative nature of the alcohol.

Chapter 16

Tinder Conk *(Fomes fomentarius)*

Common names: Hoof Fungus, Amadou (French), Iceman Polypore, Touchwood, Tsuriganetabe (Japan), Surgeon's Fungus   (PHOTOGRAPHS ON PAGE 80)

The Tinder Conk has always been common in Northeastern forests—indeed, in hardwood forests throughout temperate zones across the globe—though it usually escapes notice by those who pass it on daily walks in the woods. This all changed in 1992 with the discovery of Ötzi, the Iceman. The Tinder Conk is one of two mushrooms found with the mummified body of the Iceman, who was carrying a leather satchel filled with a significant quantity of pounded Amadou felt, along with two Birch Polypores (*Piptoporus betulinus*) carried on leather thongs around his neck. Anthropologists went into a frenzy of theorizing: What use was the Iceman making of these mushrooms? One argument was that he might have used the Tinder fungus as an antibiotic poultice for his wounds (Poder, 2005). Certainly he would have used the Amadou felt for starting fires.

Tinder Conk has a long history of use as tinder to catch a spark from flint and start a fire. It was dried and pounded into a fibrous felt used for tinder and also to carry the spark of a fire between camps. The felt, also called Amadou, was used in the days of flintlock guns to catch the spark from the flint and hold the light until the gunpowder ignited (Stamets, 2002). Historically and at present, Amadou felt is used in fly-fishing; apparently it has no equal as a drying agent for a wet, slimy fly fresh out of the fish's mouth.

Description

The Tinder Conk is a hoof-shaped (often taller than wide), sessile fruiting body of one to six inches in diameter, growing broadly attached to trunk or branch of a deciduous tree. At times the conks will grow along the underside of a projecting branch and the spore-bearing surface will be fully cylindrical. The conk is somewhat variable in color, from pale gray to buff-gray to almost charcoal, with darker shades on the older portions of the mushroom. The younger layers on the lower extremities of the conk are the palest. Resembling the rings of a clamshell, the concentric layers represent periods, not years, of growth. The conk's upper surface is smooth, with a very hard crust. The underside pore surface is somewhat concave, starting out as white with every new period of growth but quickly turning buff-gray to brown with maturity. The individual pores are tiny, three to four per millimeter, and quite long. The spore print is white.

Occurrence and Habitat

The Tinder Conk is found almost exclusively on hardwoods; in northern New England, it is frequently found fruiting on live or dead standing trees as well as on downed logs and major limbs of birches, maples, beech, and, less frequently, oaks and other hardwoods. The conks are perennial, adding new layers of growth several times a year following extended wet periods. The fruiting body is present year-round, though active growth happens only in warmer months. The conks do not generally grow for many seasons on species of paper or gray birch, as the wood decomposes quickly, resulting in conks smaller than those found on yellow birch, beech, or maples. The conks are also small on species of poplar, or aspen, whose soft wood decomposes quickly.

Ecological Information

This fungus is weakly parasitic and strongly saprobic, rotting the heartwood of the host and, while not killing the tree, markedly weakening the wood. Tinder Conk is most commonly found on dying or dead trees or the dead branches of living trees. Occasionally it will be found on the trunk of an otherwise healthy-looking tree at the site of a wound or a branch scar, which creates an opening through the bark and into the heartwood of the living tree. The Tinder Conk is called a parasite because of this growth on the dead heartwood of a living tree. Along with other wood-rotters, *Fomes* plays a major role in quietly decomposing the massive amounts of organic tissue comprising trees, recycling the carbon and major nutrients bound up in the dead wood.

Edibility

The hard, woody texture makes *Fomes* inedible.

Look-alikes

Several species of the genus *Phellinus,* notably *P. igniarius,* superficially resemble Tinder Conk but with a less pronounced hoof shape and a more pronounced, almost black, cracked upper surface and darker pore surface. The Artist's Conk, *Ganoderma applanatum,* is pale and more shelflike, and its interior flesh and tubes are whitish. The Red-belted Polypore, *Fomitopsis pinicola,* has whitish interior flesh and cream-colored tubes but a dark, almost black, upper surface with a more or less prominent reddish band on the forward edge.

Toxicity
The Tinder Conk is not known to be toxic.

Folk or Traditional Medicinal Uses
The absorbent qualities of the pounded Amadou felt, coupled with antibacterial properties, make it ideal for dressing wounds, and the native peoples of North America, Europe, and Asia used the pounded fruiting body to stop bleeding and as a physical covering on open wounds. We do not know whether native North Americans were aware of this fungus's anti-infection attributes, but in Europe, Amadou was so highly regarded as a styptic that it was given the common name Surgeon's Fungus (Hobbs, 1995).

In Europe, the long use of *Fomes* as tinder is well recorded, with the name Amadou used not only for the fruiting body but also for the finished pounded felt. Felt used for tinder is treated with lime or saltpeter to enhance its ability to catch a spark. In regions of Hungary, a variety of common names for this mushroom allude to its use as tinder and as a material for hats and other ornamental clothing accessories. One name, *zsidobu* (Jew's skin), likely refers to the fact that some Jewish traders sold the tinder felt door-to-door (Gyozo, 2005).

Across much of northern and eastern Europe, tindering—the collecting and processing of Amadou—was a significant pastime, and even an industry to supply the tinder needs of town and city. The felt was used also in the manufacture of hats, cloths, net bags, and other objects, and by shipbuilders as caulking between the planks of ships. The industry had collapsed by the end of the nineteenth century as other resources replaced the materials made from the Tinder Conk and mass-produced matches became available (Gyozo, 2005). Today, tindering is still practiced as a folk art in a few rural localities in central and eastern Europe.

The Khanty peoples of Siberia apparently use *Fomes fomentarius* as a way to expel evil ghosts and as a purification aid at funerals (Roussel et al., 2002).

Current Medicinal Uses
The Tinder Conk is used as a tonic and immune stimulator due to the action of the polysaccharides on the immune system. No clinical trials involving humans are known. In China, it is used for digestive needs and to treat several forms of cancer (Hobbs, 1995).

Several products including Tinder Conk are sold as immune boosters. They contain either extracts or tinctures of Amadou fruiting bodies, or dehydrated mycelium from culture on grain or in fermentation vats.

Areas of Research

Despite its long, traditional use as a medicinal mushroom, we have only begun to study the potential compounds and medicinal uses of this fungus.

Anti-inflammatory and pain control: A recent examination of the anti-inflammatory and pain-management potential of *Fomes fomentarius,* using rats, showed that the extract of the mushroom significantly reduced inflammation and appeared to reduce the pain response (Park et al., 2004). It was effective by inhibiting the production of some of the cell components that trigger inflammation, such as nitric oxide, TNF-alpha, and prostaglandin E-2 in the immune system macrophages.

Antitumor: In a study where *F. fomentarius* mycelia were grown in fermentation culture, the polysaccharide component of the culture broth demonstrated a direct growth-inhibiting effect on human gastric cancer cells (Chen et. al., 2008),

Antimicrobial: Amadou has been shown to inhibit growth of the bacteria *Pseudomonas aeruginosis* and *Serratia marcescens,* two common pathogens that cause human illness. In addition, extracts from Amadou are able to slow the growth of *Bacillus subtilis* (Suay et al., 2000). Hot-water decoctions of Amadou show strong antiviral properties (Stamets, 2002).

Active Components

Polysaccharides with immunostimulating and antitumor effect
Ergosterol peroxides
Antiviral and antibacterial extracts
Extracellular antimicrobial metabolites

Collection and Preservation

The Tinder Conk is found on the sides of trees and logs throughout the year. For use as a medicinal mushroom, collect the conks only when they are actively growing and producing spores; in the northeast, that is from June through October. A quick look at the pore surface will tell you whether the conk is in active growth. The pores should look fresh and evenly buff-tan. Do not collect dead conks for medicinal purposes. After the fruiting body dies, it is prone to attack by the molds and bacteria that are normally inhibited by its chemical armor.

The conk is generally easily removed from the tree by a sharp blow with the heel of the palm or the blunt end of a hatchet. On a living tree, take care not to damage the tree when chopping off the conk.

The conks are best preserved by drying. A sunny windowsill is ideal, as the ultraviolet light converts the mushroom's ergosterols to Vitamin D. Large conks are more easily dried if chopped in half. Dry conks can be stored in a closed container or a large plastic bag.

Preparation and Use

For home use, the medicinal components of Tinder Conks are collected using a hot-water extraction from the fruiting bodies, as described below. More recently, commercial extracts have been made from mycelium grown on grain or in liquid-culture vats. Ground-up fruiting bodies can be taken in capsule form, but the medicinal benefits are much more accessible through extractions made by hot-water decoction and/or alcohol. This mushroom is commonly used in mixed preparations with other medicinal mushrooms as an immunomodulator.

Amadou broth: Given the very hard texture of the Tinder Conk, it needs to be broken into smaller pieces in order to extract the medicinal components. A hatchet or stout cleaver is quite effective. Place the small pieces of mushroom in a pot, add enough cool water to cover them, and bring to a boil. Simmer the mushrooms for at least an hour—more is better—adding water if the level falls below the tops of the mushrooms.

A mixed-conk immune broth can be prepared using several woody polypore species in combination. In New England, likely candidates to share the pot will include the Red-belted Polypore, the Artist's Conk, the Birch Polypore, Reishi, and Chaga, It is easy to make this broth in bulk and freeze it in ice cube trays. Pop a mini–mushroom immune-sicle into a cup of boiling water for a daily dose. Be warned: The broth can be quite bitter if Reishi, Artist's Conk, or Birch Polypore are included. The terpenes in these mushrooms are good for you, but not always tasty!

Appendixes

Making a Double-Extraction Mushroom Tincture

Tincturing is a method of using alcohol to extract a desired group of medicinal components from an herb or mushroom. Many of the best-known medicinal mushrooms contain valuable terpenes and other factions that are soluble only in alcohol.

At its simplest, tincturing involves chopping or grinding the source material as finely as possible, covering it with ethyl (grain) alcohol, and allowing the mixture to macerate, or steep, for two weeks or more. At the end of the steeping period, the liquid tincture is strained from the solids (called the marc).

Some of the most desirable mushroom constituents are *not* soluble in alcohol, however. Almost all of the mushrooms addressed in this book contain medicinally desirable glucans and related polysaccharides that are water-soluble. They are best extracted by decoction, defined as the use of hot or boiling water to extract and concentrate desired components from a plant or mushroom. Here we use simmering water to break down the cell walls and increase the availability of the glucans.

If you are primarily interested in glucans, use a decoction to release and concentrate the polysaccharides and then freeze the broth in ice cube trays for dosed use. (Alternatively, cook up the mushrooms and enjoy the flavor as part of your regular diet.) Mushrooms best extracted using a decoction include Maitake, Oyster, and Turkey Tail. Comb Tooth, when used as an immune booster alone, also should be prepared by decoction. Alcohol can be added to the finished decoction as a preservative.

To take advantage of the *full* range of medicinal properties mushrooms represent, you want to extract both their alcohol-soluble and their water-soluble compounds. Double extraction involves first making a simple alcohol tincture, then a hot-water decoction, and finally blending the two together in the proper ratio. Mushroom species best extracted using the double tincture method include Reishi, Chaga, Artist's Conk, Birch Polypore, and Red-Belted Polypore.

The process of double extraction is not overly complex, but it does require attention to detail and a clear understanding of the concentration of alcohol in both the initial alcohol menstrum and in the final product. Because the ethyl alcohol is used not only for extraction of medicinal components but also as a preservative, it is vital that the alcohol concentration of the finished tincture be 20 percent or higher. I generally aim for 25 percent, allowing a little room for error.

Through trial and error I have concluded that the alcohol tincturing should be the first step, followed by the hot-water decoction of the remaining marc.

Ingredients Needed

Dried mushrooms, chopped or ground as finely as possible
Grain alcohol (ethanol) or vodka (100 proof or higher)
Spring water or distilled water

Medicinal components can be extracted from fresh mushrooms; however, using fresh material makes it more challenging to know the alcohol concentration of the final tincture, due to the uncertain water content of fresh fungi. Therefore, these directions call for dried mushrooms.

The type of alcohol is important because the concentration, or proof, of the alcohol determines the volume of decoction liquid (water) needed to achieve an alcohol concentration of 25 percent in the finished product. Pure, 200 proof (100 percent) ethanol is ideal but often hard to obtain without a special state-issued permit. Most liquor stores stock, or can order, 190 proof (95%) alcohol, sold under such trade names as Everclear . Many home tincture makers use 100 proof (50% alcohol) vodka or brandy. The important thing is to be certain of the proof of the liquor used.

Organic vodka and alcohol are also available, if you desire.

Equipment Needed

Stainless steel or enameled cooking pot or a slow cooker (e.g., Crock Pot)
Cheesecloth
Glass jars with clean, tight lids
Liquid measuring cup with clearly marked graduations
Chef's thermometer with probe (or candy thermometer)—optional

Step 1—Alcohol Extraction

Begin by reducing the mushrooms into pieces as small as possible by chopping, grinding, grating, or otherwise abusing the integrity of the dried fruiting bodies. This is relatively easy with dried Maitake and much more challenging with Chaga or Artist's Conk. Consider an old-fashioned meat grinder for the tougher mushrooms.

Place the finely reduced mushrooms into a glass jar and cover completely with alcohol. Be sure none of the mushroom is exposed to air. Close the jar tightly. Place it in a cupboard or closet well away from direct sunlight and shake or stir the steeping tincture every few days, adding alcohol as needed to keep the solids covered. Allow the mixture to macerate for at least two weeks; many herbalists suggest a month or one lunar cycle.

To reclaim the alcohol and its precious dissolved cargo, drain it through a strainer lined with several layers of cheesecloth, then gather the cheesecloth into a sack and vigorously squeeze out as much additional liquid as possible from the mushroom marc. **Reserve both tincture and marc!**

Very efficient commercial tincture presses are available, but for home use, cheesecloth and strong wrists make a good substitute. Plan on retrieving about two thirds of your original alcohol volume if you press your tinctured mushrooms using the cheesecloth method. Store this initial alcohol tincture in a labeled glass jar while you complete the second step of the double-extraction process.

Step 2—Hot-water Decoction

Place the strained marc in your enamel pot or slow cooker, cover with enough water to completely submerge the marc, and cook, uncovered, for two or more hours at just under boiling (190–200 degrees F). For the more woody species, or when using coarsely chopped pieces, simmer overnight. Allow the volume to reduce, but keep the mushrooms covered by adding water, if necessary.

Cool and again strain and squeeze the marc, reserving the liquid decoction. Some people repeat the decoction process with a second batch of water to retrieve the maximum level of polysaccharides, a step I sometimes take with Maitake or Turkey Tails.

Step 3—Mixing the Finished Tincture

Measure the volume of your two liquid extracts. You now have a decoction of _____ ounces and an initial alcohol tincture of ___ ounces. Your desired end product is a 75/25 tincture: 75 percent water and 25 percent alcohol. Here is where it is important to slow down and write out your equations, since it is easy to get confused.

Your initial tincture has a known alcohol content based upon the proof of the alcohol you used. For example, if you used 100 proof vodka (50 percent alcohol), and ended up with 12 ounces of pressed extract, half of that volume (6 ounces) is pure alcohol. Those 6 ounces of pure alcohol need to constitute 25 percent of the total volume of the finished tincture. Therefore the finished tincture will amount to 24 ounces, made up of 6 ounces of alcohol and 6 ounces of water (from the initial alcohol extraction) plus 12 ounces of the decoction:

$$\left(\begin{array}{c}\text{6 oz alcohol + 6 oz water}\\ \text{alcohol extraction}\end{array}\right) + \begin{array}{c}\text{12 ounces}\\ \text{decoction}\end{array} = \begin{array}{c}\text{24 ounces}\\ \text{of final tincture}\end{array}$$

If, in this example, your hot-water decoction yielded more than 12 ounces, you would need to reduce the volume to 12 ounces by further simmering before adding it into the tincture. Alternatively, you could use only 12 ounces of your decoction and save the rest for broth, but that would result in less total polysaccharide content in the finished tincture.

Calculating the proportion of pure alcohol to water is relatively simple when you are using 100 proof alcohol—and even easier if you are able to use pure, 200 proof alcohol. If you are using liquor with a different alcohol percentage, you will need to do some math.

Expressed mathematically, the formula for a finished tincture with 25% alcohol content looks like this:

$$A + B + C = 4A$$

Where:

A= Volume of pure alcohol. Calculated as volume of initial ethanol extraction x % concentration of the alcohol used.

B = Volume of water in the alcohol extraction. Calculated as volume of initial ethanol extraction – A.

C = Volume of decoction.

4A = the maximum volume of the finished tincture achieved by adding the right volume of decoction.

For a second example, let's assume you start out with 190 proof alcohol and your initial tincture process again yields 12 ounces. That initial tincture would be 95% alcohol, and your equation for determining the amount of decoction to add will use the following values for A and B:

$$(12 \times .95) + (12 - 11) + C = 4A$$

or,

$$11 \text{ oz} + 1 \text{ oz} + C = 44 \text{ oz, so } C = 32 \text{ oz}$$

For A, 95% of 12 is 11.4. (I have rounded this down to 11 ounces. Whenever you calculate the volume of total alcohol and have to round off the result, round down.) The desired final amount of tincture is 4 x 11, or 44 ounces, and therefore you would need to add 32 ounces [C] of decoction to the 12 ounces of initial tincture [A + B] to yield a total of 44 ounces.

When you have a corrected volume of decoction cooled to room temperature, pour it into a jar of sufficient volume to contain the finished product and add the initial tincture to it. The alcohol in the tincture may cause some of the polysaccharides to come out of solution, and they will settle to the bottom of the container over time. Stir or gently shake the tincture before transferring to smaller bottles or before each use to ensure fair distribution of this valuable part of the tincture. I generally pour the tincture into two-ounce, amber colored, eye-dropper bottles for daily use. Store the finished tincture in glass in a dark cupboard. Be sure you label your tincture with the mushroom used, concentration of alcohol, and the date completed. Properly made and stored, tinctures will last for several years.

I advocate the use of mixed mushroom tinctures for diverse, broad immune stimulation. I recommend that individual mushroom tinctures be made separately and blended later. This gives you the maximum flexibility in deciding the mix of mushrooms you use and the relative concentrations of each tincture in a blend. My favorite general immune tonic blend incorporates Chaga, Maitake, Reishi, and Turkey Tail. I take two full droppers (½ teaspoon) most mornings in a cup of hot water. In winter I add additional Chaga to the blend as a respiratory protector.

Take the time needed to work through to a good understanding of the process before making your first batch of tincture. Preparing a tincture from mushrooms involves obtaining raw ingredients, preparation time and skills, and acute attention to volume and concentration calculations. Not everyone may want to tackle this hands-on process. Alternatively, commercially prepared tinctures are available, including a line of tinctures made by the author.

Glossary

acquired immunity: An immune response developed over time in response to an antigen that triggers the production of antibodies specific to that antigen.

antibody: Immune system proteins that identify and neutralize foreign objects such as bacteria and viruses. Each type of antibody possesses a highly variable protein tip that corresponds to a specific antigen and acts only against that one. Antibodies are found circulating in the body or can be rapidly produced by triggered memory cells.

antigen: Anything that acts within the body to trigger an immune reaction—most commonly, malignant cells, viruses, bacteria, or fragments of these microbes, or an allergic trigger, such as pollen.

antimutagenic: Something that protects the cells against genetic mutation from such mutagens as radiation, certain chemicals, or some viruses.

antioxidant: A substance that reduces oxidative damage such as that caused by free radicals, or that acts to counteract the damaging effects of oxygen.

apoptosis, or **programmed cell death:** A programmed sequence of events that leads to the destruction of an old, unhealthy, cancerous, or otherwise undesirable cell in the body. Apoptosis plays a crucial role in eliminating unhealthy cells without damaging healthy cells.

B-cell, or **B-lymphocyte:** A type of white blood cell (lymphocyte) responsible for the production of antibodies; a major player in humoral immune response.

cytotoxic: Referring to a substance or an immune cell that is directly damaging to a cell or a microbe.

dendritic cell (DC): A type of white blood cell, generally located in areas of high microbe infiltration, that acts to break down microbes and transport antigen to B-lymphocytes to trigger broader immune response. Part of the early detection-and-response process of the immune system.

ergosterol: A form of steroid alcohol, produced by fungus, that has the same role as cholesterol in mammals. Ergosterol is also known as Provitamin D2 and is easily converted to Vitamin D.

fraction: A set of chemicals sharing common separation characteristics. An example would be a group of polysaccharides sharing a similar molecular weight and soluble in alcohol, as opposed to water soluble. Most liquors are distillate fractions of a fermentation process.

functional food: A food, food ingredient, or modified food consumed as part of a normal diet and defined by the federal Institute of Medicine as "those foods that encompass potentially healthful products, including any modified food or ingredient that may provide a health benefit beyond the traditional nutrients it contains."

hematopoiesis: The production of blood cells. In the human body, blood is made by hematopoietic stem cells in the bone marrow.

hypha (*pl.* **hyphae**): The basic vegetative unit of most larger fungi, composed of thread-like, elongated tissue one cell wide, with cells added on to elongate the thread. Hyphae are the basic feeding structures of fungi; in more complex clustering, they form the transport, food storage, and structural building blocks of fungal tissue.

hyphal knots: A thickening of the mycelium into the pinhead, or primordium, that will become a mushroom fruiting body.

immunoceutical: Referring to a substance, generally classified as a form of dietary supplement with immunomodulator action.

immunomodulator: A compound, drug, or dietary supplement capable of bringing the immune system into balance or maintaining its homeostasis through the up-regulation or down-regulation of specific aspects of immunity.

immunotherapy: Use of a variety of techniques to trigger a desired immune response directed toward a specific goal. Used primarily as a means to address cancer, though standard vaccines are a form of immunotherapy.

innate immunity: Elements of the immune system that are present from birth and do not rely on the triggering action of antigens and the development of antibodies. Includes the skin and mucous membranes, saliva and tears, elevated temperature, and macrophages and NK cells.

interferons: cytokines; a group of small proteins produced by immune and other cells in the body, that act to inhibit viral replication. Also released in response to cancer growth and acting to stimulate broad immune response.

lymphocyte: A class of white blood cells forming a vital part of the immune system of vertebrate animals. They are roughly classified by their size and their function.

macrophage: A type of large white blood cell matured from a monocyte that destroys invasive organisms or malignant cells and acts as a scavenger of dead and broken cells or other particles. Also helps to trigger a broader immune response to invasive organisms or cancers.

memory cells: A specific type of matured B-cell produced in the wake of an infection and carrying an antigen recognition code. Memory cells persist in the body for years and are able to rapidly convert to plasma cells and trigger antibody production if the infection antigen is reintroduced to the body.

monocyte: A type of white blood cell made in the bone marrow and thought of as immature. Monocytes leave the marrow, circulate in the blood, and come to rest in a variety of tissues, where they mature into different forms of macrophages.

mutagen: A substance or energy capable of causing the alteration of a gene and triggering a mutation.

mycelium (*pl.* **mycelia**): An organized network or colony of the vegetative hyphae of a fungus colonizing its environment. The mycelium is the feeding and transporting function of a fungus, absorbing nutrients from the environment and moving them to where they are needed.

mycophagy: The practice of eating mushrooms.

mycorrhizal: A mutual relationship between a fungus and plant; usually symbiotic, where the fungus acts as an extension of the root system of the plant, bringing water and nutrients from the surrounding soil, and the plant shares some of its photosynthesis-produced sugars with the fungus.

natural killer (NK) cell: Vital components of the innate immune system, NK cells are white blood cells that move freely throughout the body, concentrating in areas that have a high degree of contact with the outside world. They destroy foreign cells on contact and can trigger a broader immune response.

nutraceutical: Referring to a dietary supplement intended to have a health-promoting effect.

phagocyte: A large white blood cell designed to swallow and digest an invading organism, malignant cell, or particle.

plasma cell: A large cell that matures from a B-cell in response to infection and is responsible for the manufacture of antibodies, which are made at a rate of up to three thousand per second.

polypore: A fungus in which the fruiting body bears its spores in a fine network of tubes (pores) beneath the cap, often referring to a leathery or woody fungus with pores.

saprobe, or **saprobic**: An organism that derives its energy by decaying dead organic matter, usually dead plant tissue, and releasing the mineral nutrients for recycling.

sclerotium (*pl.* **sclerotia**): A fungal energy-storage body, made up of hyphae, to store the food energy of the fungus until the appropriate conditions exist to form a fruiting body.

stem cell: Found in the bone marrow, these cells produce red and white blood cells. Used generally to refer to a line of cells able to reproduce and differentiate into a diverse range of specialized cells.

T-cell, or **T-lymphocyte**: A class of white blood cell that plays a major role in the identification and destruction of unhealthy or malignant body cells, or foreign bodies such as bacteria or viruses.

terpene: A very large and diverse class of organic hydrocarbons made primarily by plants and fungi. Considered secondary compounds, i.e., not actively involved in feeding or cell growth, they often play a role in defending the organism from predation.

tonic: A substance that, when ingested, improves the tone of the body: a restorative agent or influence.

Traditional Chinese Medicine (TCM): A range of traditional medical practices and philosophies that view illness as resulting from imbalance of energy systems in the body rather than simply being caused by outside forces or pathogens.

triterpenes: A class of terpenes composed of variations on six connected rings of isoprene. These include sterols and a host of related organic chemicals with a diverse array of bioactive functions, including antimicrobial, anti-inflammatory, and directly antitumor.

Tumor necrosis factor: Referring to a class of cytokines with a significant role in the induction of apoptosis, or programmed cell death, of tumors or other unwanted or invasive cells.

white blood cells: Also known as leukocytes, these are the basic cells of a functioning immune system, which act to protect the body from infection, malignant cells, and foreign bodies. Found in several major types throughout the body, they originate in the bone marrow.

References

Journals

Ambach, W., and E. Ambach. 1992. Austria: Tyrol's Ice-Man. *Lancet* 339, issue 8807, June 13, 1992.

Babitskaya, V.G., et al. 2002. Melanin complex from medicinal mushroom *Inonotus obliquus* (Pers.: Fr.) Pilat (Chaga). *International Journal of Medicinal Mushrooms* 4: 139–45.

Berger, A., et al. 2004. Cholesterol-lowering properties of *Ganoderma lucidum* in vitro, ex vivo, and in hamsters and minipigs. *Lipids in Health and Disease* 3: 2.

Bisko, Nina A., et. al. 2005. Antioxidant and gene protective effects of medicinal mushrooms *Inonotus obliquus* and *Phellinus robustus*. *International Journal of Medicinal Mushrooms* 7 (3): 388.

Boa, Eric. 2004. Wild Edible Fungi: A Global Overview of Their Use and Importance to People. FAO *Non-Wood Forest Products Report* no. 17. ISBN 9251051577, retrieved from http://www.fao.org/docrep/007/y5489e/y5489e00.htm#TopOfPage 2008-3-2.

Bobek, P., L. Ozdin, and S. Galbavy. 1998. Dose and time-dependent hypocholesterolemic effect of Oyster Mushroom (*Pleurotus ostreatus*) in rats. *Nutrition* 14 (3): 282–86.

Bobek, P., and S. Galbavy. 2001. Effect of pleuran (beta-glucan from *Pleurotus ostreatus*) on the antioxidant status of the organism and on dimethylhydrazine-induced precancerous lesions in rat colon. *British Journal of Biomedical Science* 58 (3): 164–68.

Buchanan, P. K. 2001. A taxonomic overview of the genus *Ganoderma* with special reference to species of medicinal and neutraceutical importance. *Proceedings of the International. Symposium Ganoderma Science*, Aukland. 27–29.

Bukhman, V.M., et al. 2007. Preparation and biological properties of basidiomycete aqueous extracts and their mycelial compositions. *Antibiot Khimioter* 52 (1–2): 4–9.

Cha, J.Y., et al. 2005. Hypoglycemic and antioxidative effects of fermented Chaga Mushroom (*Inonotus obliquus*) on streptozotocin-induced diabetic rats. *Journal of Life Science* 15 (5): 809–18.

Chan, W.K., et al. 2008. *Ganoderma lucidum* polysaccharides can induce human monocyte leukemia cells into dendritic cells with immuno-stimulatory function. *Journal of Hematology and Oncology*. Published online July 21.

Chang, S.T., and J.A. Buswell. 1996. Mushroom neutraceuticals. *World Journal of Microbiology and Biotechnology* 12 (5): 473–76.

Chen, W., et al. 2008. Optimization for the production of exopolysaccharide from *Fomes fomentarius* in submerged culture and its antitumor effect in vitro. *Bioresource Technology* 99 (8): 3187–94.

Cheng, J.J., et al. 2008. Properties and biological functions of polysaccharides and ethanolic extracts isolated from medicinal fungus *Fomitopsis pinicola*. *Process Biochemistry* 43 (8): 829–83.

Choi, DuBok, et al. 2008. Effects of *Fomitopsis pinicola* extracts on antioxidant and antitumor activities. *Biotechnology and Bioprocess Engineering* 12 (5): 516–24.

Compendium of Materia Medica, A.D. 1590, vol. 28, pp.19–21. Reprint. Beijing: China Press.

Daba, A.S. 2005. Hypocholesterolemic effect of the Oyster Mushroom, *Pleurotus ostreatus* (Jacq.:Fr.) P. Kumm. and its isolated polysaccharides. *International Journal of Medicinal Mushrooms* 7 (3): 394-95.

Dendritic cell. In *Wikipedia, The Free Encyclopedia*. Retrieved 18:03, 2008-11-24, from http://en.wikipedia.org/w/index.php?title=Dendritic_cell&oldid=252719128.

Dong, Q., et al. A β-d-glucan isolated from the fruiting bodies of *Hericium erinaceus* and its aqueous conformation. *Carbohydrate Research* 341 (6): 791–95.

Eiznhamer, D.A., and Z.O. Xu. 2004. Betulinic acid: a promising anticancer candidate. *Drugs* 7 (4): 359–73.

Fan, L., et al. 2006. Advances in mushroom research in the last decade. *Food Technology and Biotechnology* 44 (3): 303–311.

Filip, G.M., et al. 2004. Technical note: Artificial inoculation of decay fungi into Douglas fir with rifle or shotgun to produce wildlife trees in western Oregon. *Western Journal of Applied Forestry* 19 (3): 211–15.

Fisher, M., and L.X. Yang. 2002. Anticancer effects and mechanisms of polysaccharide-K (PSK): implications of cancer immunotherapy. *Anticancer Research* 22 (3): 1737–54.

Fukushimam, M., et al. 2001. Cholesterol-lowering effects of Maitake (*Grifola frondosa*) fiber, Shiitake (*Lentinus edodes*) fiber, and Enokitake (*Flammulina velutipes*) fiber in rats. *Experimental Biology and Medicine* 226 (8): 758–65.

Fuller, R., P. Buchanan, and M. Roberts. 2005. Medicinal uses of fungi by New Zealand Maori people. *International Journal of Medicinal Mushrooms* 7 (3): 402.

Glauco, S., et al. Safety of Maitake D-fraction on healthy patients. *Alternative and Complementary Therapies* 10 (4): 228–30.

Gonzales-Angulo, A.M., F. Morqles-Vasquez, and G.N. Hortybagyi. 2007. Overview of resistance to systemic therapy in patients with breast cancer. *Advances in Experimental and Medical Biology* 608: 1–22.

Gorbunova, I.A., N.B. Perova, and T.B. Teplyakova. 2005. Medicinal mushrooms of southwest Siberia. *International Journal of Medicinal Mushrooms* 7: 403–4.

Gu, C.Q., et al. 2007. Isolation, identification and function of a novel anti–HSV-1 protein from *Grifola frondosa*. *Antiviral Research* 75(3): 250–7.

Gu, C.Q., J. Li, and F.H. Chao. 2006. Inhibition of hepatitis B virus by D-fraction from *Grifola frondosa*: synergistic effect of combination with interferon-alpha in HepG2 2.2.15. *Antiviral Research* 72 (2): 162–5.

Gyozo, Z. 2005. Tinder Polypore and Birch Polypore in Hungarian popular tradition. *Mycological-Ethnomycological Journal* 3: (3) 51–61. (Translated from the Hungarian.)

Hayakawa, K., et al. 1997. Effect of Krestin as adjuvant treatment following radical radiotherapy in non-small cell cancer patients. *Cancer Detection and Prevention* 21 (1): 71–7. (Clinical study, abstract.)

Hobbs, C.L. 1995. *Medicinal Mushrooms: An Exploration of Tradition, Healing and Culture*. Santa Cruz, Calif.: Botanica Press.

Hong, L., M. Xun, and W. Wutong. 2007. Anti-diabetic effect of an alpha-glucan from fruit body of maitake (*Grifola frondosa*) on KK-Ay mice. *Journal of Pharmacy and Pharmacology* 59 (4): 575–82.

Hossain, S., et al. 2003. Dietary mushroom (*Pleurotus ostreatus*) ameliorates atherogenic lipid in hypercholesterolemic rats. *Clinical and Experimental Pharmacology and Physiology* 30: 470–75.

Huss, M.J., et al. 2002. The efficacy of inoculating fungi into conifer trees to promote cavity excavation by woodpeckers in managed forests in western Washington. USDA Forest Service General Technical Report PSW-GTR-181.

Hwang, H.S., et al. 2008. Production of extracellular polysaccharides by submerged mycelial culture of *Laetiporus sulphureus var. miniatus* and their insulinotropic properties. *Applied Microbiology and Biotechnology* 78 (3): 419–29.

Ikekawa, T. 2005. Cancer risk reduction by intake of mushrooms and clinical studies on EEM. *International Journal of Medicinal Mushrooms* 7 (3): 347.

Jeong, Y.T., et al. 2008. *Ganoderma applanatum*: a promising mushroom for antitumor and immunomodulating activity. *Phytother Research* 22 (5): 614–19.

Jiang, J., et al. 2004. *Ganoderma lucidum* suppresses growth of breast cancer cells through the inhibition of Akt/NF-kappaB signaling. *Nutrition and Cancer* 49 (2): 209–16.

Jiménez-Medina, E., et al. The immunomodulator PSK induces in vitro cytotoxic activity in tumour cell lines via arrest of cell cycle and induction of apoptosis. *BMC Cancer.* 24 March 2008.

Jose, N., T.A. Ajith, and K.K. Jananrdhanan. 2002. Antioxidant, anti-inflammatory, and antitumor activities of culinary-medicinal mushroom *Pleurotus pulmonarius* (Fr.) Qul. (Agaricomycetideae). *International Journal of Medicinal Mushrooms* 4 (4): 329.

Kahlos, K., et al. 1996. Preliminary tests of antiviral activity of two *Inonotus obliquus* strains. *Filoterapia* 67 (4): 344–47.

Kanazawa, M., et al. 2004. Effect of PSK on the maturation of dendritic cells derived from human peripheral blood monocytes. *Immunonology Letters* 91 (2): 229–38.

Kawagishi, H. Ph.D., et al. 2002. The inducer of the synthesis of nerve growth factor from Lion's Mane *(Hericium erinaceus)*. *Explore* 11 (4). Can be accessed online at www.explorepub.com/article/kawagishi_11_4.html.

Keller, A.C., M.P. Maillard, and K. Hostettmann. 1996. Antimicrobial steroids from the fungus *Fomitopsis pinicola*. *Phytochemistry* 41(4) : 1041–46.

Kenmoku, H., et al. 2002. Erinacine Q, a new erinacine from *Hericium erinaceum*, and its biosynthetic route to erinacine C in the basidiomycete. *Bioscience, Biotechnology, and Biochemistry* 66 (3): 571–75.

Kidd, P. M. 2000. The use of mushroom glucans and proteoglycans in cancer treatment. *Alternative Medicine Review* 5 (1): 4–27.

Kim, H.G., et al. 2007. Ethanol extract of *Inonotus obliquus* inhibits lypopolysaccharide-induced inflammation in RAW 264.7 macrophage cells. *Journal of Medicinal Food* 10 (1): 80–89.

Kim, Y.O., et al. 2006. Anti-cancer effect and structural characterization of endo-polysaccharide from cultivated mycelia of *Inonotus obliquus*. *Life Science* 79 (1): 72–80.

Kobori, M., et al. 2007. Ergosterol peroxide from an edible mushroom suppresses inflammatory response in RAW 264.7 macrophages and growth of HT29 colon adenocarcenoma cells. *British Journal of Pharmacology* 150 (2): 209–19.

Kodama, N., K. Kiyoshi, and H. Nanba. 2002. Can Maitake MD-fraction aid cancer patients? *Alternative Medicine Review* 7 (3): 236–39.

Kodama, N., et al. 2005. Enhancement of cytotoxicity of NK cells by D-fraction, a polysaccharide from *Grifola frondosa*. *Oncology Reports* 13 (3): 497–502.

Kodama, N,, et al. 2005. Maitake D-fraction enhances antitumor effects and reduces immunosuppression by mitomycin-C in tumor-bearing mice. *Nutrition* 21 (5): 624–29.

Kolotushkina, E.V., et al. 2003. The influence of *Hericium erinaceus* extract on myelination process in vitro. *Fiziolohichny zjurnal* 49 (1): 38–45.

Konno, S., et. al. 2001. A possible hypoglycaemic effect of Maitake mushroom on type 2 diabetic patients. *Diabetic Medicine* 18 (12): 1010.

Konno, S. 2007. Effect of various natural products on growth of bladder cancer cells: two promising mushroom extracts. *Alternative Medicine Review* 12 (1): 63–68.

Krieger, L.C.C. 1936. *The Mushroom Handbook.* Reprint. New York: Dover Publications, 1967.

Kudo, S., et al. 2002. Effectiveness of immunochemotherapy with PSK,a protein-bound polysaccharidem in colorectal cancer and changes of cancer marker. *Oncology Reports* 9 (3): 635–38 (Clinical study, abstract).

Kuo, M. February 2004. *Ganoderma tsugae.* Retrieved from the MushroomExpert.Com Web site: http://www.mushroomexpert.com/ganoderma_tsugae.html.

Lakahmi, B., et al. 2004. Antimutagenic activity of methanolic extract of culinary-medicinal Oyster Mushroom (*Pleurotus ostreatus*; strain florida) and its protective effect against benzol (a) pyrene-induced hepatic damages. *International Journal of Medicinal Mushrooms* 6 (2): 139–49.

Lee, S.H., et al. 2006. Constituents from the fruiting bodies of *Ganoderma applanatum* and their aldose reductase inhibitory activity. *Archives of Pharmacal Research* 29 (6): 479–83.

Lee, S.I., et al. 2007. Antihyperglycemic effect of *Fomitopsis pinicola* extracts in streptozo-tocin-induced diabetic rats. *Journal of Medicinal Foods* 11 (3): 518–524.

Lin, H., et al. 2004. Maitake beta-glucan MD-fraction enhances bone marrow colony formation and reduces doxorubicin toxicity in vitro. *International Immunopharma-cology* 4 (1): 91–99.

Lin, H., et al. 2007. Enhancement of umbilical cord blood cell hematopoiesis by mai-take beta-glucan is mediated by granulocyte colony-stimulating factor production. *Clinical and Vaccine Immunology* 14 (1): 21–27.

Lindequest, U., et al. 2005. The pharmacological potential of mushrooms. *eCAM* 2 (3): 285–99.

Lo, H.C., T.H. Hsu, and C.Y.Chen. 2008. Submerged culture mycelium and broth of *Gri-fola frondosa* improve glycemic responses in diabetic rats. *American Journal of Chinese Medicine* 36 (2): 265–85.

Lull, C., H. Wichers, and H. Savelkoul. 2005. Anti-inflamatory and immunomodulating properties of fungal metabolites. *Mediators of Inflammation* 2: 63–80.

Masuda, Y., et al. 2008. Inhibitory effect of MD-fraction on tumor metastasis: involve-ment of NK cell activation and suppression of intercellular adhesion molecule (ICAM)-1 expression in lung vascular endothelial cells. *Biological and Pharmceutical Bulletin* 31 (6): 1104–8.

Mayell, M. 2001. Maitake extracts and their therapeutic potential: a review. *Alternative Medicine Review* 6 (1): 48–60.

Miura, N.N., et al. 2002. Blood clearance of (1,3)-beta-D-glucan in MRL Ipr-Ipr mice. *FEMS Immunology and Medical Microbiology* 13 (1): 51–57.

Mizuno, T., et al. 1983. Studies on the host-mediated antitumor polysaccharides, 5: Chemical structure and antitumor activity of a water-soluble glucan isolated from Tsugasaruno-koshikake, the fruit body of *Fomitopsis pinicola*. Shizuoka University (Japan) *Bulletin of Faculty of Agriculture* 32: 29–40.

Moncalvo, J.M. 2005. Molecular systemics of *Ganoderma:* What is Reishi? *International Journal of Medicinal Mushrooms* 7 (3): 353–54.

Moran, M. 2003. The cost of bringing new drugs to market rising rapidly. *Psychiatric News* 38 (15): 25.

Mori, K., et al. 2008. Improving effects of the mushroom Yamabushitake (*Hericium eri-naceus*) on mild cognitive impairment: a double-blind placebo-controlled clinical trial. *Phytother Research* 23 (3): 367–72.

Mori, K., et al. 2008. Nerve growth factor-inducing activity of *Hericium erinaceus* in 1321N1 human astrocytoma cells. *Biological and Pharmceutical Bulletin* 31 (9): 1727–32.

Nakajima, Y., Y. Sato, and T. Komishi. 2007. Antioxidant small phenolic ingredients in

Inonotus obliquus (persoon) Pilat (Chaga). *Chemical and Pharmaceutical Bulletin* (Toyoko) 55 (8): 1222–26.

Nakata, T., et al. 2006. Structure determination of inonotus oxides A & B and in vivo anti-tumor promoting activity of inotodiol from the sclerotia of *Inonotus obliquus*. *Bioorganic and Medicinal Chemistry* 15(1): 257–64.

Nakatsugawa, M., et al. 2003. *Hericium erinaceum* (yamabushitake) extract-induced acute respiratory distress syndrome monitored by serum surfactant proteins. *Internal Medicine* 42 (12): 1219–22.

Namba, H. 1995. Results of a non-controlled clinical study for various cancer patients using Maitake D-fraction. *Explore!* 6 (5).

Namba, H., and K. Kubo. 1997. Effect of Maitake D-fraction on cancer prevention. *Annals of the New York Academy of Sciences* 833: 204–7.

Ohno, N. 2005. Structural diversity and physiological function of beta-glucans. *International Journal of Medicinal Mushrooms* 7(1 & 2): 167–73.

Ohwada, S., et al. 2004. Adjuvant immunochemotherapy with oral Tegafur/Uracil plus PSK in patients with stage 2 or 3 colorectal cancer: a randomized controlled study. *British Journal of Cancer* 91 (6): 1220-21.

Park, E., K.I. Jeon, and B.H. Byun. 2005. Ethanol extract of *Inonotus obliquus* shows antigenotoxic effect on hydrogen peroxide induced DNA damage in human lymphocytes. *Cancer Prevention Research* 10: 54–55.

Park, K.Y., et al. 2004. Chaga mushroom extract inhibits oxidative DNA damage in human lymphocytes as assessed by comet assay. *Biofactors* 21: 109–12.

Park, Y.M., et al. 2004. Anti-inflammatory and anti-nociceptive effects of methanol extract of *Fomes fomentarius*. *Biological and Pharmaceutical Bulletin* 27 (10): 1588–93.

Park, Y.M., et al. 2005. In vivo and in vitro anti-inflammatory and anti-nociceptive effects of the methanol extract of *Inonotus obliquus*. *Journal of Ethnopharmacology* 101 (1–3): 120–28.

Pilz, D., et al. 2003. Ecology and management of comercially harvested Chanterelle mushrooms. USDA Forest Service General Technical Report PNW-GTR-576.

Pisha, E., et al. 1995. Discovery of betulinic acid as a selective inhibitor of human melanoma that functions by induction of apoptosis. *Nature Medicine* 1: 1046–51.

Poder, R. 2005. The Ice Man's fungi: facts and mysteries. *International Journal of Medicinal Mushrooms* 7: 57–58.

Preuss, H.G., et al. 2007. Enhanced insulin-hypoglycemic activity in rats consuming a specific glycoprotein extracted from maitake mushroom. *Molecular and Cellular Biochemistry* 306 (1–2): 105–13.

Roussel, B., et al. 2002. History of the therapeutic uses of Tinder Polypore (*Fomes fomentarius*) (in French). *Revue d'histoire de la pharmacie* (Paris) 50 (336): 599–614.

Saito, T., et al. 1998. Erinacine E as a kappa opioid receptor agonist and its new analogs from a basidiomycete, *Hericium ramosum*. *Journal of Antibioics* (Tokyo) 51 (11): 983–90.

Schar, D. *Grifola frondosa*: A possible addition to the Materia Medica. Planet Botanic. www.planetbotanic.com. Accessed on 6-01-08.

Silva, D., et al. 2003. Biologic activity of spores and dried powder from *Ganoderma lucidum* for the inhibition of highly invasive human breast and prostate cancer cells. *eCAM* 9 (40): 491–97.

Silva, D. 2004. Cellular and physiogical effects of *Ganoderma lucidum* (Reishi). *Mini-Reviews in Medical Chemistry* 4: 873–79.

Smith, J.E., N. Rowan, and R. Sullivan. 2002. Medicinal mushrooms: their therapeutic properties and current medical usage with special emphasis on cancer treatments. (Special report commissioned by Cancer Research UK). Available online at http://sci.cancerresearchuk.org/labs/med_mush/med_mush.html.

Smith, J.E., and R. Sullivan. 2004. The western approach to medicinal mushrooms. *KMITL Science and Technology* 4(1). Available online at http://www.kmitl.ac.th/ejkmitl/vol4no1/Mushrooms.pdf.

Son, C.G., et al. 2006. Macrophage activation and nitric oxide production by water soluble components of *Hericium erinaceum*. *International Immunopharmacology* 6 (8): 1363–69.

Stamets, P. 2002. Novel antimicrobials from mushrooms. *HerbalGram* 54: 28–33.

Stamets, P., 2005. *Mycelium Running: How Mushrooms Can Help Save the World*. Berkeley: Ten Speed Press.

Storm, 2004. The usefulness of Polypores in primitive fire making. *Mushroom, the Journal of Wild Mushrooms*. www.mushroomthejournal.com.

Suay, I., et al. 2000. Screening of basidiomycetes for antimicrobial activities. *Antonie van Leeuwenhoek* 78: 129–39.

Taji, S., et al. 2008. Lanostane-type triterpenoids from the sclerotia of *Inonotus obliquus* possessing anti-tumor promoting activity. *European Journal of Medicinal Chemistry* 43 (11): 2373–79.

Takeda, K., and K. Okumura. 2004. CAM and NK cells. *eCAM* 1(1): 17–27. http://ecam.oxfordjournals.org/cgi/content/full/1/1/17. Accessed online on 11-04-08.

Tanaka, H., et al. 2001. Three-year follow-up study of allergy in workers in a mushroom factory. *American Journal of Respiratory and Critical Care Medicine* 95 (12): 943–48.

Tang, Y.M., R. Yu, and J.M. Pezzuto. 2003. Betulinic acid-induced programmed cell death in human melanoma cells involves mitogen-activated protein kinase activation. *Clinical Cancer Research* 9: 2866–75.

U.S. Dept. of Health and Human Services. 2003. *Understanding the Immune System: How It Works*. NIH publication 03-5423. Available online at http://www.niaid.nih.gov/Publications/immune/the_immune_system.pdf.

Volk, T. 2001. *Fomes fomentarius*. Tom Volk's Fungus of the Month for December, 2001. Accessed on 6-01-08 at http://botit.botany.wisc.edu/toms_fungi/dec2001.html.

Von Kemami Wangun, H. 2006. "Isolation, Structure Elucidation and Evaluation of Anti-inflammatory and Anti-infectious Activities of Fungal Metabolites." Doctoral dissertation, Freidrich-Schiller University, Jena, Germany. Accessed online at www.db-thueringen.de/servlets/Derivate-10437/KemaniWagun/Dissertation.pdf.

Wang, G., W. Tang, and R.R. Bidigare. 2005. "Terpenoids as therapeutic drugs and pharmaceutical agents." In *Natural Products: Drug Discovery and Therapeutic Medicine*. Totowa, N.J.: Humana Press.

Wang, J.C., et al. 2001. Antitumor and immunoenhancing activities of polysaccharide from culture broth of *Hericium spp. Kaohsiung Journal of Medical Sciences* 17 (9): 461–67.

Wang, J.C., et al. 2001. Antimutagenicity of extracts of *Hericium erinaceus. Kaohsiung Journal of Medical Sciences* 17 (5): 230–38.

Wang, L., et al. 2008. Oral administration of submerged cultivated *Grifola frondosa* enhances phagocytic activity in normal mice. *Journal of Pharmacy and Pharmacology* 60 (2): 237–43.

Books on Medicinal Mushrooms

Chang, S.T., and P.G. Miles. 2004. *Mushrooms: Cultivation, Nutritional Value, Medicinal Effect and Environmental Effect.* 2d. ed. CRC Press.

Halpern, G.M., and A.H. Miller. 2002. *Medicinal Mushrooms: Ancient Remedies for Modern Ailments.* New York: H. Evans and Co.

Hobbs, C.L. 1995. *Medicinal Mushrooms: An Exploration of Tradition, Healing and Culture.* Santa Cruz: Botanica Press.

Stamets, Paul. 2002. *Mycomedicinals: An Informational Treatise on Mushrooms.* Olympia: Mycomedia.

Mushroom Identification and Information

Arora, D. 1986. *Mushrooms Demystified.* Berkeley: Ten Speed Press.

Besette, A.E., A.R. Besette, and D.W. Fischer. 1997. *Mushrooms of Northeastern North America.* Syracuse University Press.

Lincoff, G. 1981. *The Audubon Society Field Guide to North American Mushrooms.* New York: Alfred A. Knopf.

Phillips, R. *Mushrooms and Other Fungi of North America.* 2005. Firefly Books.

Web Site Resources

www.mskcc.org/mskcc/html/11570.cfm A site hosted and maintained by Memorial Sloan- Kettering Cancer Center and devoted to information and research supporting the use of herbs and medicinal mushrooms. Designed for information directed at the lay person or medical professional. Fairly conservative and medical model in scope and focus.

www.healing-mushrooms.net/about-this-website This informative and very well referenced site is the ongoing work of Robert Sasata. His goal is to review and reference medicinal information on more than 900 species of mushrooms. At this point he has more than 150, and by the time you read this the list will undoubtedly have grown significantly.

http://sci.cancerresearchuk.org/labs/med_mush/med_mush.html Smith, J. E., N.J. Rowan, and R Sullivan. 2000. *Medicinal mushrooms: their therapeutic properties and current medical usage with special emphasis on cancer treatments.* This is a great monograph devoted to an in-depth review of mushroom use, research, and potential regarding cancer treatment.

Index

www.ingramcontent.com/pod-product-compliance
Lightning Source LLC
Chambersburg PA
CBHW041258040426
42334CB00028BA/3072